THE Pilates

DIRECTORY

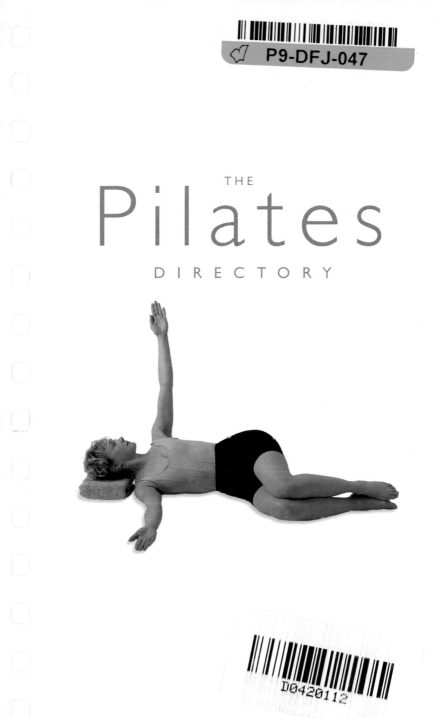

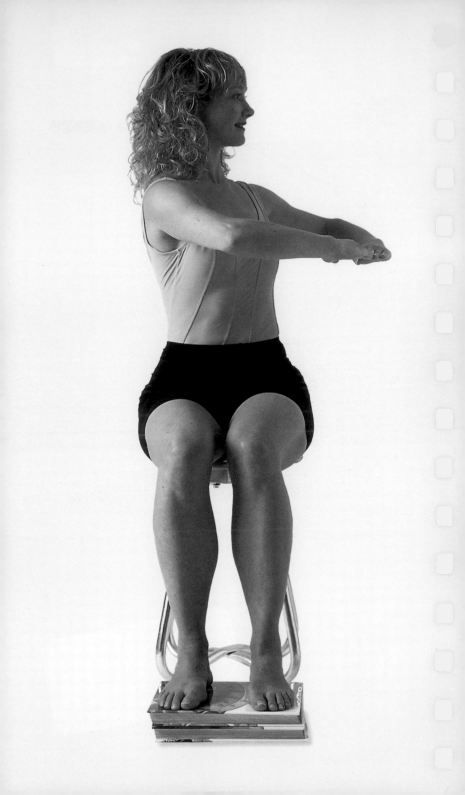

THE
Pilates
DIRECTORY

Alan Herdman

CHARTWELL
BOOKS, INC.

First published in 2004 by
Chartwell Books Inc.
A Division of Book Sales Inc.
114 Northfield Avenue
Edison, New Jersey 08837

ISBN: 0-7858-1796-4

Note from the publisher
Information given in this book is not intended to be
taken as a replacement for medical advice. Any person
with a condition requiring medical attention should
consult a qualified medical practitioner or therapist.

This book was conceived, designed, and produced by
THE IVY PRESS LIMITED
The Old Candlemakers
Lewes, East Sussex BN7 2NZ

CREATIVE DIRECTOR: Peter Bridgewater
PUBLISHER: Sophie Collins
EDITORIAL DIRECTOR: Steve Luck
SENIOR PROJECT EDITOR: Caroline Earle
DESIGN MANAGER: Tony Seddon
DESIGNER: Alistair Plumb
ARTWORK ASSISTANT: Joanna Clinch
PHOTOGRAPHY: Paul Forrester
PICTURE RESEARCH: Liz Eddison
ILLUSTRATIONS: Michael Courtney

Printed and bound in China

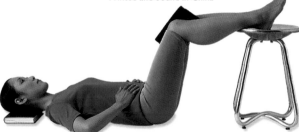

contents

Introduction

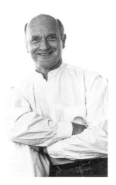

Alan Herdman
The author established the
first Pilates studio in the
UK in 1970 and now runs
several all over the world.

What is the secret of Pilates? Actors and dancers swear by it. Physical therapists and osteopaths regularly refer patients to it. People who've switched between different kinds of exercise and keep-fit routines, without achieving the effects they wanted, breathe a sigh of relief when they discover Pilates. Why is it so popular? The answer is that Pilates is extremely effective. Within weeks of starting, you will have better posture, toned muscles, a flatter stomach, and looser, more flexible joints. Some people even claim to get taller as their spine is stretched and straightened. Joseph Pilates, who designed the Pilates system in the early 20th century, claimed: "In 10 sessions you will feel the difference, in 20 you will see the difference, and in 30 you'll have a whole new body." Now if that doesn't motivate you, what will?

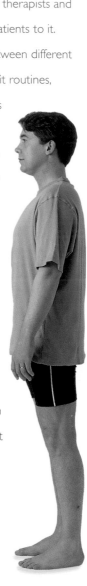

Lifelong benefits
Pilates teaches your body how to
move correctly even when you are
not exercising.

Pilates works in a completely different way from circuit training, gym workouts, and weight machines. Their effect is to increase the bulk of the strongest muscles of the body, shortening and tightening them in the process. Pilates exercises lengthen and strengthen all the muscles, down to the deepest core, while making sure that the body is correctly balanced and aligned. Those who think a workout hasn't been effective if they don't feel exhausted and aching should consider that muscle soreness is caused by lactic acid buildup, improper stretching, and even tearing of muscle fiber. In Pilates, the message is quality, not quantity: muscles are worked precisely and efficiently but no more than is necessary. You should never feel pain either during or after a Pilates session.

Breathing
Pilates breathing techniques can relieve stress and increase energy, by delivering more oxygen to your muscles.

This book explains from scratch, lesson by lesson, everything you need to know to establish your own Pilates routine. Before starting any exercise, you are taught to make sure that your body is perfectly aligned. You learn how to isolate individual muscle groups and work them without putting strain on any other area. Once you understand a movement, you will find that your muscles "remember" the correct positions next time you try. As the muscles are stretched and elongated, the mobility of the joints increases and the stress on them reduces, so regular Pilates exercises are very successful at relieving niggling joint pains and sciatica, and can have miraculous effects on people with injuries and severely weakened areas. If you have a history of injury, or spinal or joint problems, you should consult your specialist before starting this course, but be assured that, performed correctly, the movements are completely safe. Recommendations and alternative methods for those who have difficulty doing a specific exercise are given where appropriate. If you are pregnant or have just had a baby, read pages 190–95 for some extra advice.

Pilates is a great antidote to the stresses of everyday life. You won't be able to think about anything else during a Pilates session apart from the movements that you are making and the sensations in your body. After exercising, you won't ache or feel tired. Your joints will be looser and there is a sense of calm that comes from the flowing rhythm of the exercises.

Joseph Pilates taught that the key to achieving change is believing that you can do it. You have already taken one step in the right direction by deciding to read this book. Relax, enjoy, and look forward to the new body that awaits you. It's going to be easier than you think.

Alignment
You will learn how to check that every part of the body is aligned correctly before you begin an exercise.

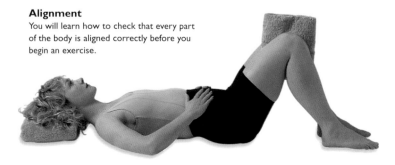

Joseph Pilates

Born in 1880 in Düsseldorf, Germany, Joseph Pilates was a sickly child. During his early years, he suffered from asthma, rickets, and rheumatic fever, which left him with a stunted bone structure and twisted limbs. Rather than accept the limitations of his body, he decided to overcome them and he worked systematically and tirelessly, developing a series of exercises to correct his disabilities. These formed the basis of his

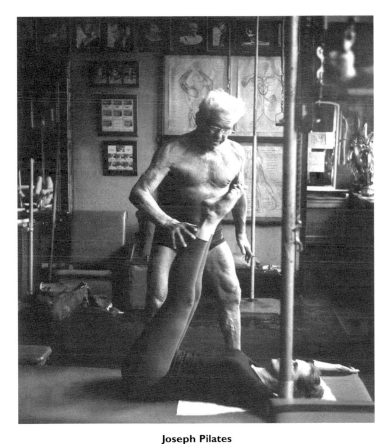

Joseph Pilates
The early mechanisms he devised using bedsprings were the prototypes of the machines you can find in Pilates studios today.

renowned "matwork exercises," which he called "The Art of Contrology."
In 1912, Pilates went to England, where he worked in a variety of
physical roles: as a boxer, a self-defense instructor, and even a circus
performer. On the outbreak of the World War I, and along with other
Germans in the United Kingdom, he was interned as an "enemy alien,"
first in Lancaster and then on the Isle of Man. While working in a
hospital on the Isle of Man, he helped some of the injured patients to
regain their mobility as they lay in bed: with bedsprings attached to the
bed-frame, he supported their damaged limbs so they could move the
area safely and keep their muscles toned.

Pilates' fame began to spread after the people he was treating
proved strong enough to survive a devastating influenza epidemic
that swept Britain in 1918. In 1926, he moved to New York, where
celebrity clients such as dancer Martha Graham and choreographer
George Balanchine became regulars at his studio. Before his death in
1967, Pilates had trained some other instructors to teach his system.
Foremost among them were Bob Fitzgerald and Carola Trier, from
whom I learned the method in the late 1960s.

I established the first Pilates studio in London in 1970, and have
since established several others around the world, where we teach
clients and train new instructors. Over the years, I have continued to
develop and adapt the exercises, in order to deal with the problems
and body types clients bring to me. There is no doubt that if Joseph
Pilates were still around today, he would have developed his method
further to deal with the stresses and strains of 21st-century life,
such as working on computers.

The Pilates Principles

The exercise system in this book is my own, but it is firmly based on the principles Joseph Pilates invented a century ago. Here are the basics:

1 Concentration

When you start Pilates, there's a lot to think about. Sometimes it feels as though you're being asked to rub your stomach, pat your head, and keep breathing to a set rhythm, all at the same time. The key is to focus your thoughts on the area you are exercising, paying attention and noticing how your muscles respond.

2 Control

There should be no sloppy, involuntary, jerky, or hurried movements in Pilates. Once you learn how to control the muscles, you will be able to perform the movements in a smooth, fluid way throughout the range in which each muscle is capable of moving.

3 Core stability

Many Pilates exercises are dedicated to strengthening the torso and building a strong core that will support the rest of the body. You'll find references to "core stability" in almost every lesson in this book, because it is fundamental for aligning and balancing the body while protecting the spine.

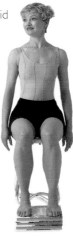

Slow and steady
The exercises are performed slowly and smoothly.

4 Breathing

Taking a full breath in and then expelling it completely is beneficial in many ways. Using your breathing correctly lets you perform the Pilates exercises more efficiently and gain maximum benefit from them.

5 Precision

When doing Pilates exercises, it is important that you perform every single direction to the letter. If you are just a half-inch out of the correct alignment, the exercise will be much less effective.

6 Visualization

The mind should work in conjunction with the body during Pilates exercises, and the lessons suggest some visual images to help you imagine what you should be doing. Once you can see the correct movement in your mind's eye, the body will follow.

7 Integration

All of these principles should come together when you perform an exercise, so that you feel your body as a whole, even when you are working on one particular muscle group.

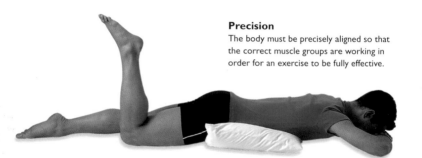

Precision
The body must be precisely aligned so that the correct muscle groups are working in order for an exercise to be fully effective.

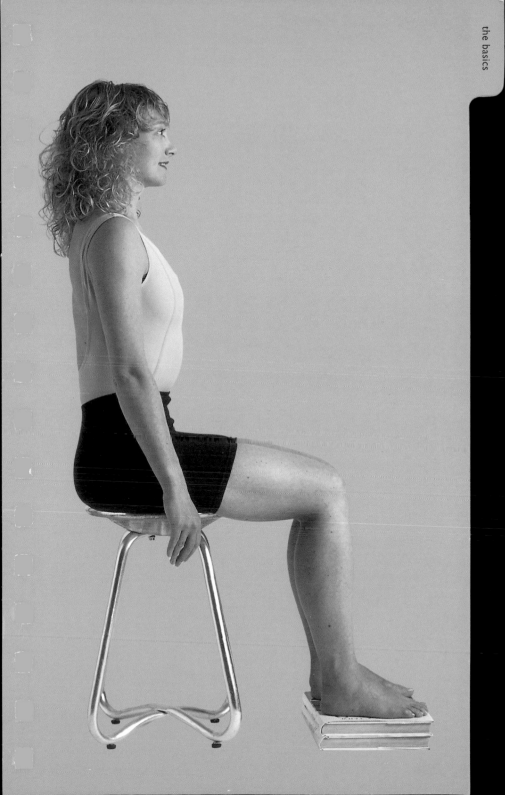

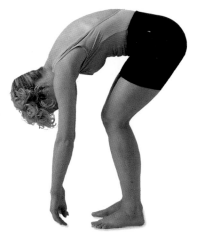

The Basics

Before you attempt a Pilates exercise, you will have to check your posture carefully. Are your feet level with your hips? Are your shoulders relaxed downward? Are you comfortable or does any area feel strained? You'll need to learn about the breathing patterns that work with, rather than against the movements. And you'll require a basic understanding of the muscle groups so that you can establish a particular way of moving in your "muscle memory." Then you put all the basics together. Feel your spine lengthening and visualize your muscles getting longer as the fibers stretch to their limit but not beyond. Think of the oxygen flowing into your system with the in breath and the carbon dioxide being expelled as you breathe out. Sounds complicated? It's not really. There will be a moment, quite early on, when you suddenly "get it"—and after that, there's no looking back.

Posture

The human body is designed to be perfectly balanced and held in position by gravity when you stand straight with your feet directly below your hips. It should be possible to run a plumb line from just behind the ear, through the shoulder joint, hip joint, and knee joint, hitting the floor just below the ankle joint. The weight of the body should be evenly distributed on the feet.

Poor posture can be caused by inherited conditions, disease, or injury, but for most people it is the result of bad habits repeated over and over again. When schoolchildren carry a bag on one shoulder day after day, they are developing a tendency to favor one side and, as adults, it won't feel "right" to carry a bag on the other shoulder. Children who are taller than their contemporaries can develop a tendency to stoop. Women who wear high heels that tilt them forward develop a tendency to lean backward for balance, forcing the lower back to arch. In each of these cases, it is the repetition year after year that sets the action. Muscles tighten and shorten in the area, eventually pulling bones and joints out of alignment, and that's when the pain and dysfunction set in.

The intention of this lesson is not to give you instant perfect posture before you proceed any further in the book. Habits that your body has

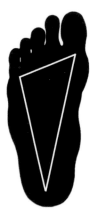

Foot triangle
When standing, imagine a triangle with the apex at the front of the heel (just below the ankle joint) and the base across the pads of the foot before the toe joints; your weight should be supported on this triangle.

learned over the years will take some time to unlearn. However, it is important to be aware of any weaknesses and postural problems before you start so that you can consciously correct your position and arrange all your joints in alignment before each exercise. It may feel "wrong" at first, as you unlearn your bad habits, but stick with it. Remember: If you are just half an inch out of alignment, the exercise will be much less effective.

Perhaps you think your posture is pretty good already? That may be the case, but when they start Pilates some people are surprised to discover asymmetries they weren't aware of before. You may find, for example, that you can manage an exercise easily on one side but it's much harder on the other.

Stand in front of a full-length mirror to do a self-assessment test. Wear comfortable clothing that enables you to see your outline, and remove your shoes. Stand with your feet slightly apart, in line with your hip joints, and run through the checklist on pages 16–17.

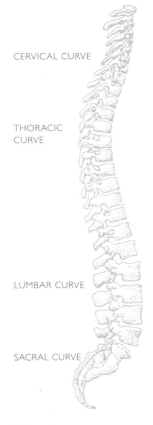

CERVICAL CURVE

THORACIC CURVE

LUMBAR CURVE

SACRAL CURVE

The spine
The vertebrae of the spine form four natural curves. Pilates exercises can help correct any distortion of this natural alignment.

Self-Assessment

Facing sideways

● Would a plumb line dropped from behind your ear pass through the shoulder, hip, and knee joints and hit the floor just behind the ankle?

● Does your chin jut out or tilt upward? If so, you will be pulling your neck out of alignment. As you look straight ahead, your chin should be level and pulled slightly backward.

● Are your shoulders hunched forward, or are they pulled rigidly back? Raise your shoulders to your ears and let them drop back naturally into position.

● Does your upper back curl forward? *See kyphosis, page 20.*

● Is the arch of your back pronounced? Do your bottom and/or stomach stick out? Read the section on lordosis on page 19–20.

Facing forward

● Are your shoulders level or is one slightly higher than the other? This could be the case if you always carry bags on one side, or answer the phone with the same hand.

● Are your arms hanging loosely by your sides, with your fingers in a straight line and parallel to the fingers on the other hand? If not, this could mean you are holding one shoulder higher than the other.

OBJECTIVITY

Be as objective as possible when doing the self-assessment. Get a friend to examine you and answer the questions on your behalf. Another tip is to glance in a store window as you're passing, to check your "inadvertent posture"—the one you adopt when not in front of a mirror doing a Pilates self-assessment!

● Are your hip bones level? If not, this could indicate that one leg is slightly shorter than the other, or it could be a symptom of scoliosis (see *page 19*), but it is most likely to mean that you tend to sit with your weight leaning into one hip. See *hip problems, page 20–21*.

● Check the gap between your lower arm and your hips. Is it equal on both sides? If not, this could mean that you are prone to sitting on one hip rather than balancing your weight equally on both sides.

● Are your knees facing straight forward or are they turned inward or outward? *See the advice on knee pain on page 21.*

● Is your weight balanced equally on the heels, outsides of your feet, balls of your feet, and toes? *See the triangle illustration on page 14.*

● Are you tensing any muscles as you stand here? This is a dead giveaway that something is not in true alignment.

Posture
Pilates can help correct many
common postural faults.

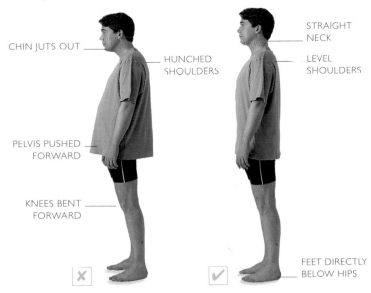

CHIN JUTS OUT

HUNCHED
SHOULDERS

PELVIS PUSHED
FORWARD

KNEES BENT
FORWARD

STRAIGHT
NECK

LEVEL
SHOULDERS

FEET DIRECTLY
BELOW HIPS

Posture Problems

Don't despair if you have identified postural problems. Almost everyone has some, but most can be corrected and all can be alleviated through Pilates exercises. Once you learn to stretch and lengthen the muscles responsible for posture, they will hold you comfortably and effortlessly in perfect balance. It's useful to try and visualize your spine and remember the position that it should be in. Monitor it throughout your daily routine. What is happening to your spine as you sit at your computer? When you have your legs crossed? As you pick up a toddler and balance him on one hip? Or curl up on the couch to watch television? Have an awareness of your position while you are sitting and standing, and before long your body will start to obey the rules. Meanwhile, here are some of the most common postural complaints explained.

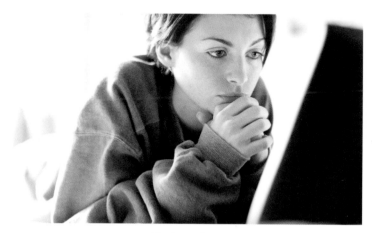

Neck tension
People who sit hunched over a desk or computer often experience neck and shoulder stiffness. It is important to design your work station so that the desk, chair, and screen are in positions that let you sit correctly.

Neck and shoulder tension

This is one of the main problems experienced by people who have desk jobs. The neck muscles are weak and the shoulder muscles tighten to compensate, until you can feel them bunched up and rock hard under the skin. The exercises in The Back section will help to release neck and shoulder tension, but it is also important to strengthen the muscles of the torso so that they hold your posture correctly. If you suffer from neck pain, it can help to support the weight of the head with a small cushion for the exercises that require you to lie on your back.

Scoliosis

In scoliosis, the spine is bent to one side in the thoracic or lumbar area, and sometimes another part of the spine curves in the opposite direction, causing an "S" shape. This condition often starts to develop in childhood: the schoolboy carrying his knapsack on one shoulder, while his bones are still developing, could be heading in this direction. Scoliosis can also result from a spinal injury or congenital abnormalities like poliomyelitis. Although there are different degrees of scoliosis, you should always seek medical advice, as it can be a very serious condition. Pilates can help, but you should book a one-to-one consultation with a qualified instructor before trying the exercises in this book.

Lordosis

The spine naturally curves inward in the lower back, and this curve is necessary for shock absorption. However, in some people the curve has become pronounced because their pelvis is out of alignment and

TAKE CARE

When you catch yourself using in a bad
postural habit, don't jerk suddenly to
correct it. Stop, breathe, and realign
naturally. The exercises on pages
22–25 will show you how.

their abdominal and gluteus
(bottom) muscles are weak.
Pronounced inward curvature
can lead to lower back pain, disk
prolapse, and even osteoarthritis.
The tightness in front of the hips can restrict walking. Pilates combats
lordosis by strengthening the stomach muscles, hamstrings, and gluteus
muscles, improving core stability. Lordosis sufferers should be careful
not to force their lower back down to the floor when lying flat on their
backs. It can help to prop a cushion under the upper back, or place
the feet up on a small box or stool.

Kyphosis

This is an excessive forward curve of the upper spine, giving a humped,
rounded appearance. It can be caused by a variety of bone and spinal
disorders, including osteoporosis. A tendency to kyphosis is created in
people who stoop as children. Bad kyphosis can restrict breathing as
the chest is slumped forward and the ribs are unable to move properly.
Pilates can help to correct kyphosis by strengthening the muscles of the
upper back. The exercises on pages 118–36 will be helpful. When lying
down, make sure that the head is well supported with a pillow.

Hip problems

If you have noticed that one hip is higher than the other, it doesn't
necessarily mean that one leg is shorter than the other. If you tend
to sit with your weight balanced one on side, or with your legs crossed,
the muscles around the waist will eventually shorten on one side,

holding the hip higher. Focusing on the exercises in the Core Stability chapter will help to lengthen the muscles and align your hips again. If you have had a hip replacement, you need to avoid movements that adduct or abduct the hip joints (move the thigh in or out in a sideways direction rather than in front of you or behind you). Seek advice from your physician before starting Pilates.

Knee pain

When the knees are habitually held in an improper position, the muscles round about them tighten to grip them in place. It is important that you keep your knees soft and never "lock" them when exercising. Gradually, through Pilates, you will learn to use the muscles of the inner thighs and buttocks instead, but in the meantime, some of the leg exercises include modifications that will avoid straining your knees. If you have had a knee replacement, seek advice from your physician before exercising.

Foot problems

There is no point in working hard to correct posture if the feet are not supporting your body weight evenly. Pilates can help to strengthen the muscles on the front of the foot and get the weight into the center. If you have problems with your feet, focus especially on the exercise on page 172.

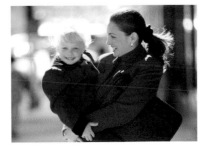

Holding one hip higher
Habitually carrying a toddler on one hip will eventually cause the muscles on one side of the waist to shorten.

Ways of Correcting Posture

Several times a day, you should stop and run through a checklist to assess your posture. Uncross your legs, then straighten your spine, draw in your stomach, and let your shoulders relax. You will instantly feel better. You should always run through a posture checklist before beginning Pilates exercises, because if there are any misalignments in your body, you will not feel the full benefits of the movements.

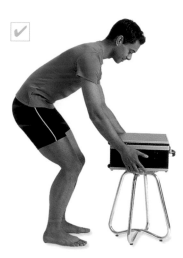

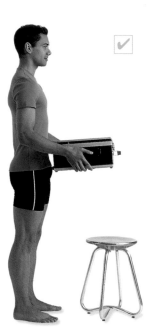

TAKE CARE

If you have to lift a heavy object, bend your knees to pick it up, then let your legs do the work. Don't ever bend from the waist, which would put strain on the lower back. Keep the object as close to you as possible while you are lifting, and never twist around while holding it.

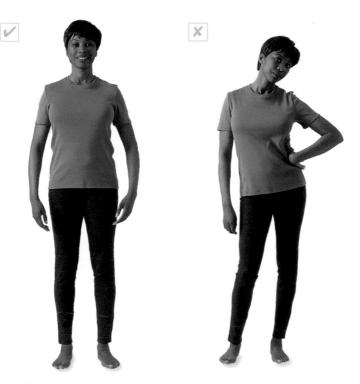

STANDING

When standing, you should maintain the alignment described on page 14. Your knees should be straight with the muscles gently engaged but not locked, and both feet should be firmly on the ground with your weight distributed equally on the triangle shapes on each side (see the diagram on page 14). If you want to bend one knee, make sure that you keep the weight evenly distributed between your feet and don't sink into the hip on one side. Keep the hips square. You should feel a slight tension in the buttocks as they support you.

A simple exercise that you can do when standing at the kitchen sink, or in line at the bank, is to gently squeeze your buttock muscles together. Breathe in, and as you breathe out, squeeze as though you are trying to touch your buttocks together. Don't squeeze too hard or grip the muscles. Relax and repeat.

SITTING

Make sure both feet are firmly on the ground. Don't cross your legs. Your back should be positioned as much into the back of the chair as possible: if the chair seat is too long, place a cushion at the base of your back. The backs of your thighs should rest on the chair and your weight should be supported on them and in your feet. Choose a chair that lets you sit with your knee joints and hip joints bent at right angles. Gently draw your stomach in and let your shoulders relax.

Spine Roll-down

The spine roll-down is a lovely stretch for the spine. Your shoulders should be relaxed and your navel should be pulled back throughout this exercise so that the abdominal muscles are doing the work and there is no strain on the back.

❶ Stand straight with your feet shoulder-distance apart. Imagine that your spine is stuck to a wall. Breathe out and gently pull your navel backward, then bend your knees slightly and peel your spine slowly off the wall from the top down. Lower your chin forward to your breastbone, then your ribs toward your hips, still keeping your lower back against the imaginary wall and letting your arms hang loosely.

❷ Breathe in halfway down, then, as you breathe out, continue to relax your upper body forward as far as it will go, softening your knees further. Don't worry if you can't touch your toes—just go as far as you can manage comfortably.

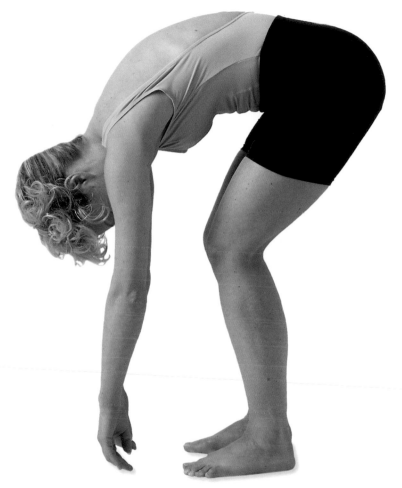

STATIC ABS—SEATED

Try this simple exercise when sitting in the office or driving a car. Sit correctly, as described on page 23, and breathe in. Then, as you breathe out, think of drawing your navel toward the back of the seat. Repeat this as often as you like.

❸ At the bottom of the roll-down, take another breath in, keeping your navel pulled back and knees bent. Breathe out and reverse the movement, peeling upward slowly and sticking your spine bit by bit back onto the imaginary wall. Lengthen the ribs away from the hips and move back to standing with a straight spine.

Questions & Answers

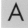 **Q** Why don't you wear sneakers to do Pilates? Wouldn't they help you to grip the floor better?

A You need to feel your feet working during Pilates and shoes might hinder this. There are a lot of nerve endings on the soles of the feet that can help you feel whether you are using them correctly, so it is best to have bare feet or wear socks. If you are on a slippery surface, place a nonstick mat underneath your feet to hold them in position.

Q When I try to do the spine roll-down, there are loud clicks and cracks in my back. Should I be worried about this?

 A Not if it doesn't hurt. Clicks don't necessarily mean that the joints are under stress; they can be perfectly natural and indicate a kind of release rather than a strain. If you experience any pain connected with clicks in your back, though, you should see a doctor.

Q I have pronounced bunions, which affect the way I walk. Instead of my feet landing firmly on the ground, they "roll" from one side to the other. Can Pilates help this?

 A Pilates can't cure bunions, but by strengthening the muscles in your feet, it can help to balance your weight more solidly across your feet. Once your balance is better, your walking will improve. Try the balance tests on pages 160–61 to see how you are progressing.

Q I'd like some tips on good posture for desk workers. I'm afraid that 40 hours a week at a computer will undo any good work I do in Pilates.

A When sitting at a computer, make sure your chair is close enough to the desk to keep your lower arms at right angles to your torso. If you have to lean forward, bend from the hips, not the lower back. Don't spend more than 20 or 30 minutes at a time in this position. Sit up and stretch, and try an exercise like the sitting lats (*see pages* 108–9).

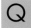 **I am very tall and since I was a child I have walked with a slight hunch. How can I "unlearn" this bad postural habit?**

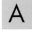 Pilates will help, by opening the upper torso and getting your body back into alignment. Monitor your posture during the day and if you find yourself hunching, stop and adjust your posture, as described on page 23.

 So should I never wear high heels again? Can't I get away with them for special occasions?

 Certainly you can wear high heels if you want to, but not for long periods of time. Make sure your shoes are a good fit and that they support your feet so you aren't straining to keep them on. If you feel unsafe in your high heels, don't wear them: Be comfortable.

 Which sleeping position is best for your spine?

You should always make sure your spine is supported on a mattress that isn't too hard or too soft. The fetal position, curled on one side, is good. A pillow should support your neck at the right height to keep the spine in a straight line. If you suffer from lower back pain, try placing a pillow between your knees when lying on your side.

 I frequently have to carry bags full of books home from the library. How should I carry them if not in a shoulder bag?

Shoulder bags are not good news. If you are carrying heavy bags of any kind, try to hold one on each side for balance. Don't lock your elbows; keep them slightly bent so as not to strain the joint. Alternatively, a small knapsack worn on your back will spread the weight more evenly.

Breathing

Most people don't breathe properly. They take short breaths from the top of their lungs and don't expel them completely when they breathe out. This means that the body's pumping system, by which oxygen is flushed into the bloodstream and carbon dioxide is flushed out, is not working efficiently. Since all the muscles in the body—including the heart—require oxygen in order to function, this is a problem that can have a knock-on effect.

There are two nerves that control breathing. One originates in the top of your spine and the other is linked to the digestive system, larynx, and heart. That's why when you take quick, shallow breaths—as we tend to do when we're stressed—you can suffer from nausea, a dry mouth, and palpitations. Learning to breathe correctly is one of the best methods of stress relief, and it can work instantly. Breathing deeply with full inhalations and exhalations is energizing. You must first hold your head, neck, and back in proper alignment. If your shoulders are slumped forward, or your chin tilted back, the airway won't be fully open and the muscles that control breathing won't be able to stretch fully.

As you breathe in, your ribs expand outward and backward and the abdominal muscles lengthen. When you breathe out, the abdominal muscles shorten, pulling the ribs downward. If this movement isn't controlled, the rib cage will slump toward the stomach and the spine will bend forward. Keeping the spine long and straight introduces an opposing force that stops the ribs from collapsing into the stomach. The upper ribs, which are attached to the spine and breast bone, should rotate slightly on the out breath, while the lower ribs move in toward the center of the body, making the chest narrower from side to side and slightly narrower from back to front. Stand in front of a mirror and check your own breathing. As you breathe in, there shouldn't be any upward movement of the shoulders or tensing of the muscles in the neck. When you breathe out, the shoulders shouldn't pull downward, your spine should stay straight, your collar bones shouldn't move, and the neck should be free of tension.

Breathing during exercise

Breathing correctly is important when doing any kind of exercise. Try this little illustration. Sit with your arms by your sides. Take a deep breath in while raising your arms above your head. Hold your breath and bring your arms down slowly, as though you are pulling them down through molasses. Now try the same movement again, but this time breathe out as you pull your arms down. This is much easier, isn't it? We have a tendency to hold our breath during exertion, but

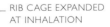

RIB CAGE EXPANDED
AT INHALATION

RIB CAGE AFTER
EXHALATION

Inspiration and expiration
When you breathe in, the rib cage moves outward and backward (solid line) and the abdominal muscles lengthen. When you breathe out, the abdominal muscles contract and pull the rib cage down (dotted lines).

this is counterproductive. Holding your breath while exercising prevents the muscles from getting the oxygen that they need and puts a strain on the chest and upper spine.

There are basic rules that govern the breathing patterns during Pilates exercises. Most importantly, it helps to breathe in through your nose and out through your mouth to fill and empty your lungs efficiently. You can breathe out for longer without tension and it's easier to control this through your mouth. There are specific breathing directions with every exercise , but generally you should breathe out on the effort part of an exercise and breathe in during preparation for the next movement.

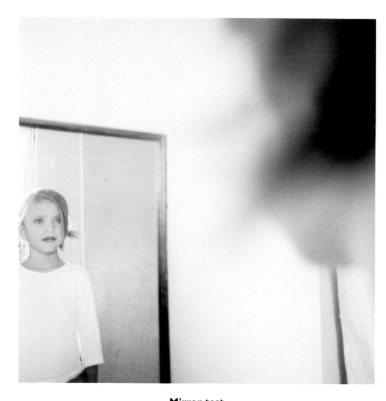

Mirror test
See if you are breathing correctly by standing in front of a mirror and checking
that your neck and shoulders don't move as you breathe.

BLOWING BUBBLES

During Pilates exercises, you have to vary the length of your outbreaths depending on the movements you are required to make at the same time. This is a simple method of learning to control the length of the outbreath, using a glass of water and a straw.

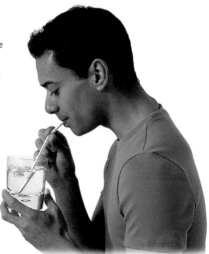

① Sit straight on a chair holding a glass of water and a straw with both hands at chest level. Breathe in through your nose to a count of four.

② Breathe out through your mouth into the straw, blowing bubbles to a count of four. Next time breathe out to a count of six, and then try eight.

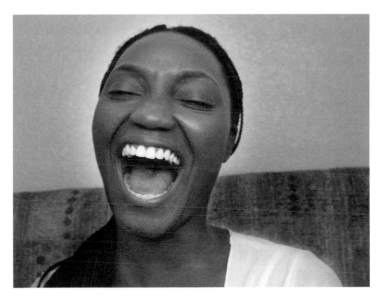

PRACTICING THE BREATHING TECHNIQUE

Whenever you have a few spare minutes during the day, do some Pilates breathing practice. Breathe in through your nose to a count of four, feeling your ribs move outward, then vary the length of the outbreath through your mouth to a count of four, six, eight, and even ten. The sooner you master the breathing technique, the better. Once it becomes second nature, you will be able to focus on the sensations in your muscles during the exercises without the distraction of having to think about your breathing as well.

Breathing Exercises

It is useful for beginners to start a Pilates session by doing some breathing exercises. As well as letting you check that you are breathing correctly by helping you to visualize the movements of your ribs, they also have a calming effect and put you in the right frame of mind.

BREATHING WITH A SCARF OR TOWEL

❶ Sit upright with your head facing forward. Take a scarf or a towel folded lengthwise and place it around your upper back, covering the area from just under your arms down to the lower part of your ribs.

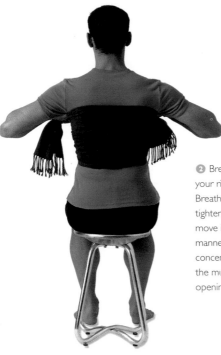

❷ Breathe in through your nose, feeling your ribs push the scarf or towel outward. Breathe out through your mouth, gently tightening the scarf, and feel the ribs move inward in a slow, controlled manner. Repeat this exercise ten times, concentrating on the movements of the muscles and the sensation of opening your chest.

SEMISUPINE

This is a variation on the last exercise. You still use the scarf or folded towel, but this time you are lying down, with your knees bent, in a common Pilates position known as "semisupine." (In the supine position, you lie on your back with your legs straight.) If you don't have a scarf or towel on hand, you can feel the same effects by pressing the backs of your hands against your ribs just underneath the armpits.

❶ Wrap the scarf or towel around your lower back. Lie on your back with your knees bent, feet placed firmly on the floor and hip-width apart. Support your head with a small cushion and relax your shoulders into the floor.

❷ Breathe in through your nose, letting your ribs push the scarf or towel outward and feeling your chest opening. Tighten the scarf as you breathe out, feeling the inward movement of your ribs. Repeat ten times.

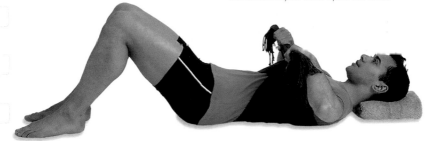

SCOOPING THE NAVEL

You will come across a similar exercise, known as static abs, on pages 51–53, which is the basic starting point for many of the Pilates exercises in this book. In the version here, you have your feet raised on a box or stool, since it can be easier to isolate the muscles this way.

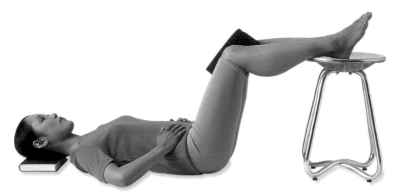

❶ Lie on your back with your knees bent and supported on a box or stool, so that your hips and your knees are bent at angles of 90°. Place a small flat cushion or rolled-up towel between your thighs to maintain the alignment of your pelvis. Place your hands on your lower abdomen. Breathe into your lungs as before, but this time let your breath go down into your abdomen.

❷ Breathe out slowly, and pull your navel toward the floor, creating a "scoop" shape. Don't squeeze your thighs together. Keep your shoulders relaxed. Repeat ten times.

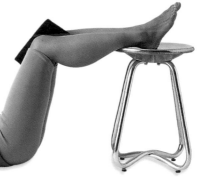

BREATHING INTO YOUR BACK

It may sound odd at first, but this is a simple and very effective method of assisting deep breathing, by opening up all the underused muscles between the ribs in your sides and in your back (the intercostal muscles).

❶ Sit upright with your head facing straight forward. Your spine should be long, your weight evenly balanced on your tailbones. Pull your navel toward your spine.

❷ Instead of breathing into your chest, try breathing into your back. Make sure you don't curve your shoulders forward or look down. Keep the shoulders soft and the spine straight. Imagine you're inflating a beachball between your shoulderblades! It may feel difficult at first, but after a few attempts your breathing will feel deeper as the muscles stretch outward. Count to five as you breathe in and five as you breathe out. If you find this difficult, just count to four. Repeat the exercise ten times.

Questions & Answers

Q When breathing out through the mouth, should I be blowing the air out?

A No; when you blow air out you are tensing the muscles and forcing it. Think of the air slowly trickling or dribbling out of your mouth. You will learn to vary the length of your exhalations depending on the rhythm of the exercise. If the movement is short, your exhalation will be quicker and if it is long, your exhalation will be slower.

Q I am asthmatic and carry a ventilator wherever I go. Will this affect my ability to do Pilates?

A Not at all. Pilates breathing is very beneficial for asthmatics, as you are strengthening the muscles and getting more breath control. You should be perfectly capable of performing the exercises, but keep your movements very slow and don't push yourself too hard.

Q I find it hard to remember the movements and breathe correctly at the same time. Can I work on the movements and add the breathing later?

A You could, but it would be hard to change your breathing patterns later once you've got into a habit. It would be much better to go slowly on some of the simpler exercises and work at them until you've got the feeling of breathing correctly.

Q I'm a smoker. Does this mean I won't be able to do Pilates breathing properly?

A It's going to make it much harder and you'll take longer to learn the breathing than nonsmokers. The best advice would be to quit smoking, but if you find this too difficult, just persevere with the breathing exercises and you'll get there in the end.

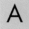 **Q** **Sometimes I feel dizzy with the breathing patterns required in exercises. What should I do?**

A If you are dizzy, this means that you are overbreathing, taking too many breaths. Keep your breath softer, cut down on the number of breaths, and slow down until you get the correct rhythm.

 Q **As a singer, I'm taught to breathe one way, in yoga they teach another way, and in Pilates a third way. Which is correct?**

A Singing teachers use different methods, but many teach pupils to breathe into the back and use the full lung capacity. So long as you are in control of your muscles and breath, you will be able to do what is needed for the discipline. Pilates breathing is correct for Pilates, yoga breathing for yoga, and the singing method is best for your singing.

Q **Which of the breathing exercises would be most useful to practice when I'm very stressed?**

A Lie on your back with your knees bent and feet firmly on the floor, supporting your head with a small cushion. Place your hands on your abdomen and rest your elbows on the floor. Breathe in slowly through the nose and out through the mouth. Repeat the exercise ten times and I guarantee this will make you feel less stressed.

Q **Why do we have to breathe out on the effort part of a Pilates exercise? I feel as though I want to breathe in.**

A If you are doing an abdominal curl and try to breathe in as you curl forward, you are moving against full lungs. If you breathe out and empty the lungs, there is more space for the movement. Blow up a long balloon, then hold the top and try to bend it in half. Now start to release the air and it will bend in half easily. Same principle!

Understanding Muscle Groups

Our bones are connected by ligaments. Joints, like the elbow, hip, and knee, enable the bones to move in relation to each other. But it's the muscles that provide the support to keep bones and joints in position and exert the forces that cause them to move. There are different levels of muscle—deep and superficial—and none of them work in isolation. The muscles that raise your left eyebrow are connected to the muscles in your little toes, via a roundabout route. Try lifting your little finger right now and look at all the subtle movements going on inside your hand and wrist.

It's a basic rule of science that for every force exerted, there must be an equal force in the opposite direction. In the body, this means that when you are contracting one set of muscles, another set will be stretching. You have already learned that a strong abdominal wall protects the spine, whereas weak abdominal muscles exert pressure on the spine. It's actually a lot more complicated than a simple backward and forward pressure. Weak muscles in one area can create a chain

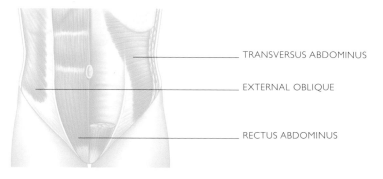

TRANSVERSUS ABDOMINUS

EXTERNAL OBLIQUE

RECTUS ABDOMINUS

reaction that affects several different parts of the body, as they tighten and tense trying to compensate for the imbalance. In Pilates, you will learn how to use all your muscles correctly in order to avoid this "snowball effect." If you ever feel a stretch in muscles apart from the ones you are exercising, stop immediately and adjust your position.

Here's an illustration. Stand straight and balanced as you were taught on page 14: Shoulders level, arms by your side, abdomen pulled in, feet directly under hips, weight distributed evenly across the feet. Pause and concentrate on how this feels. Now, put your hands on your hips and feel the changes. The pressure on your hips makes the pelvis tilt forward, your lower back arches, and your stomach sticks out. More than this, the muscles at the front of the thighs shorten to hold the pelvis in place; the weight will push you forward onto the balls of your feet; your shoulders will hunch and your neck muscles tighten to counterbalance the arch in your lower back. All from one simple action.

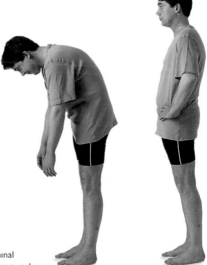

Spine roll-down
As you bend forward, your abdominal muscles contract and back muscles stretch.

Quality Versus Quantity

The best-quality movements stretch and lengthen your muscles through the range they are capable of moving but no more. You shouldn't continue repeating exercises until the muscles are exhausted; stop after the exact number of repetitions suggested and move onto another muscle group. In a balanced Pilates routine, you will use all the main muscle groups but switch continually from one to another so none of them get tired. It's also important that you don't proceed to more advanced stages of an exercise until you can perform the early stages perfectly, so you are not overtaxing the muscles.

The movements in Pilates will be much slighter and subtler than you are used to if you've ever been to an aerobics class or worked out in a gym. If there is a direction to squeeze your buttocks, it doesn't mean you should grip and tense them as hard as you can until your

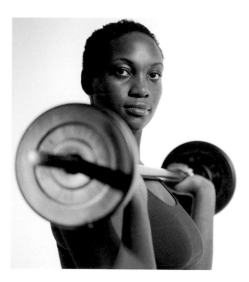

Lifting weights
If weightlifters have even a slight misalignment of muscles, they risk serious injury.

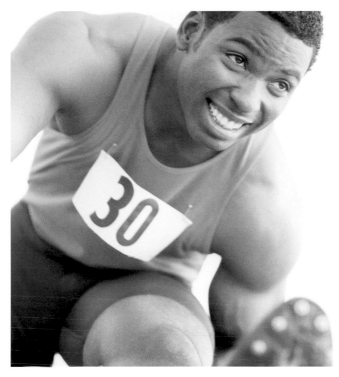

Sprinting
Some athletes build bulk in muscle groups such as the quadriceps, at the fronts
of the thighs, but they risk injury if they don't balance this by strengthening
the opposing group of muscles as well.

bottom tucks under. Instead, you should concentrate on the muscle
that runs over each of your buttock cheeks—the gluteus maximus—
and imagine pressing one side toward the other. The pressure should
be as though they are kissing each other, but no more.

Being able to visualize, to put your thoughts into the muscles you
are exercising, helps a lot. That's why, on the next pages, we will run
through the major muscle groups, explaining what each one does. As
you're reading, picture the muscles and try the movements described.
Touch them with your fingers to help to set them in your memory.

Front of the Body

There can be several muscle groups all doing roughly the same job. This is especially the case around joints, like the shoulder or hip, because they can often move in several different directions and therefore they need to be stabilized from several different angles.

STERNOCLEIDOMASTOID ❶
enables the head to bend to the side; you'll see this stand out when singers strain their voices. Bend your head gently to one side and touch the opposite side of your neck to locate this muscle.

DELTOIDS ❷
move the arms up and down and extend them to the sides. Place your left hand at the top of your right arm, just under the shoulder joint, and raise your arm outward to feel the deltoid working.

SERRATUS ANTERIOR ❸
pulls the shoulderblades forward. Place your left hand on your side under your right armpit and squeeze the right arm inward to feel this muscle in your side.

PECTORALIS MAJOR ❹
raises the arms horizontally and rotates them inward. Place your right hand in front of your left armpit and then raise your left arm to feel this muscle working.

ADDUCTORS ❺
bring the legs inward and slightly rotate them. Sit on the ground with one knee bent and the other leg extended outward. Draw the straight leg across toward the bent one to feel the adductor working.

TAKE CARE

If you have any injuries or weak areas, don't do these movements for now. Exercises that work the muscles safely will be described in the relevant chapters.

⑥ RECTUS ABDOMINUS

bends the body forward. Just curve your upper torso forward to feel this muscle, which runs all the way from the breastbone to the pubic bone.

⑦ BICEPS

bend and flex the arm and turn the hands outward. Place a hand on your upper arm and bend the arm upward from the elbow to feel them.

⑧ OBLIQUES

rotate the body and bend it to the sides. Sitting in a chair, place your hands on your sides just at the base of the ribs and turn your upper body from side to side to feel the obliques working.

⑨ TRANSVERSE ABDOMINALS

run across the abdomen in a band and are used in Pilates to pull your navel to your spine. Do it now. Breathe in and, as you breathe out, pull your lower abdomen toward the back of the chair.

⑩ QUADRICEPS

bend the knees, extend the leg, and lift it forward. Sitting on a chair, place your hand on top of your right thigh and straighten the right leg outward to feel the quadriceps.

Back of the Body

Many of the muscle groups oppose each other. Some pull the shoulderblades back while others pull them forward. Some bend the arms while others straighten them. It's important to keep these opposing groups balanced in strength to maintain the body's equilibrium.

TRAPEZIUS ❶

is a huge muscle that supports the upper back and arms. It raises the shoulders and draws the shoulderblades backward. This muscle can bunch up, causing tension in the shoulders.

RHOMBOID MAJOR ❷

rotates the shoulderblades and pulls them toward the spine. Pull your shoulderblades together to feel the rhomboids working.

INTERCOSTALS ❸

are muscles between the ribs, used in inhalation and forced exhalation. Place your left hand on the right side of your ribs and raise your right elbow. You'll feel them as the ribs open out.

LATISSIMUS DORSI ❹

keeps the shoulderblades down, pulls the arms backward, and rotates them inward. To feel the lats, lie on your front with your hands extended above your head and resting on a small towel. Your nose should be just resting on the floor. Pull the towel toward you, feeling the muscles working just under your shoulderblades.

5 TRICEPS

straighten the arms. Place the fingers of your right hand on the back of your left arm, just above the elbow joint. Bend the left arm at the elbow and as you straighten it, you should feel the triceps muscle working.

6 GLUTEUS MAXIMUS

extends and outwardly rotates the hip, extends trunk, and causes slight inward and outward movement. Squeeze your buttocks together to feel the glutes working

7 HAMSTRINGS

flex the knee, rotate it, and extend the hip. Stand up holding onto a door, then bend one leg backward from the knee and you'll feel the hamstring working in the back of your thigh.

8 GASTROCNEMIUS AND SOLEUS

flex the ankle as the foot is moving downward in walking and the gastrocnemius also flexes the knee. Place a hand on your calf, then point your toes to feel these calf muscles working.

Questions & Answers

 Q What do people mean when they say that they have "pulled" a muscle?

 A When a muscle hasn't been worked correctly, the fibers can get strained and tear. These injuries can cause bleeding into the muscle tissue and a scar is formed, which shortens the natural length of the muscle. If you follow the directions and suggested number of repetitions exactly in Pilates exercises, this won't happen.

Q If you have an injury that has weakened the muscles in one area, is it best to protect them until they heal?

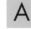 **A** Seek the advice of your specialist if you have had an injury. Sometimes it is good to work a muscle gently in order to help it to heal. Protecting an area could cause the muscles to shorten and throw the body out of balance.

Q I can understand how to use most of the external muscles, but how is it possible to locate and use the internal muscle groups?

A Don't worry about it. The internal muscles work anyway as part of the movement in Pilates exercises. All the muscle groups described in this lesson are voluntary muscles that we can consciously control, and their action works internal muscle layers at the same time.

Q What should I do if certain muscles are too strong?

A Pull back on the use of the strong muscles and work the opposing set. If you have strong quadriceps, you should work the hamstrings, and if you have strong biceps, you should work the triceps. The whole idea of the technique is creating balance so that the muscle groups all work harmoniously together.

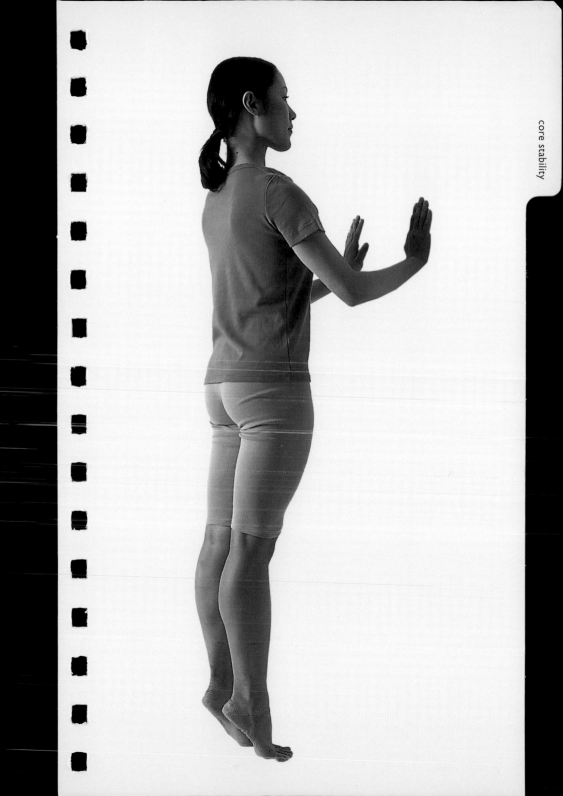

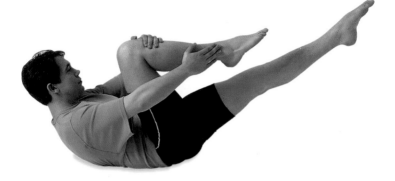

Core Stability

The muscle groups around the center of the body—in the abdomen, hips, buttocks, pelvic floor, and inner thighs all work together to keep the spine and pelvis aligned, thus promoting "core stability." They are like a kind of "girdle of strength," holding all the bones, joints, and abdominal organs in place. You will start to build your core stability from the very first time you do a Pilates exercise and follow the instruction to pull your navel toward your back. The more you practice this movement, the stronger you will get and the faster you will be able to advance to exercises that require strong core stability. If you develop an awareness of your abdominal and pelvic muscles and hold them correctly throughout your everyday life, whenever you think of it, you will build strength in them very quickly.

The Abdomen

In the first chapter, the importance of strong abdominal muscles in supporting your lumbar spine and maintaining good posture was explained. A strong abdominal wall will also hold the organs of your abdomen in the correct positions, enabling them to function to their full capacity. In particular, the coils of the lower part of the digestive system are supported properly, and this can help to alleviate digestive disorders such as constipation, flatulence, and irritable bowel syndrome. The kidneys and bladder can work more efficiently and women may find their period pains are relieved.

The muscles that we will be focusing on in this section are the transverse abdominals, which run across the area between the ribs and pelvis; the rectus abdominus, which runs vertically from the pubic bone to the breast bone, enabling us to bend forward; and the external and internal obliques, which tuck around our sides and let us do side bends and turn sideways. All three of these groups have to be strong to help provide "core stability."

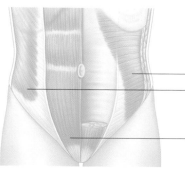

The abdominal muscles
These muscles support the torso, back, and abdominal organs.

TRANSVERSUS ABDOMINUS
EXTERNAL OBLIQUES

RECTUS ABDOMINUS

You will notice the effects of these exercises quite quickly. People report feeling that their stomach is flatter after less than ten sessions of exercising. Concentrate hard during the exercises to make sure you can feel the muscles you are working and that you aren't inadvertently stretching somewhere else. Less is more. Tiny, accurate movements are much better than larger, inaccurate ones that could put strain on other areas.

Men are especially prone to laying down fat in the abdominal area, as a "beer gut" or "love handles," and women may lose muscle tone after childbirth and start to lay down fat layers here after menopause. Pilates can be very effective in combination with a weight-loss diet, because you can focus on the areas you particularly need to trim. Flabby muscles are less responsive than lean, toned ones, because the fibers are working through layers of fat. As you work those muscles regularly, however, you will target the fat layers and help to shift them. So, overweight people should do the same exercises but put more emphasis on the areas they want to tone.

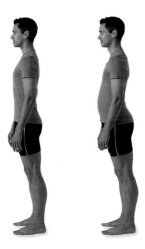

Strong abs
Note all the differences
well-toned abdominal
muscles make to posture.

Equipment and Clothing

Most of the exercises in this chapter are performed lying down. Ensure that the surface you are working on is not too hard and not too soft. A thick carpet, a rug, or a folded blanket are fine, or use an exercise mat if you have one. Wear loose, comfortable clothing, such as leggings and a T-shirt, and keep your feet bare or wear socks. Avoid belts, buttons, buckles, or anything that might constrain you. Make sure the room temperature is warm enough for comfort but not too hot. The only other props you will need for these exercises are a towel, a few different-sized cushions or pillows, and a box or a chair that is about the same height as the length of your thighs.

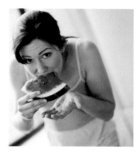

Healthy diet
Pilates will tone your muscles, but if you need to lose weight, the only way is to eat less. Cut out junk food, don't eat too late in the day, and drink lots of water.

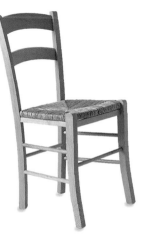

TAKE CARE
If you are pregnant, read the advice on pages 190–95. Many of the abdominal exercises in this section will be unsuitable for you.

Static Abs

This group of exercises will begin to work your abdominal muscles. It's crucial that you can do them correctly because almost every other Pilates exercise in this book will require you to pull your navel through to your back, thus engaging the abdominal muscles, before you perform a movement. Don't suck your stomach in; this creates a dip at the top of the abdomen under the ribs, while the lower abdomen protrudes.

ON ALL FOURS

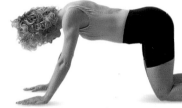

❶ Get down on your hands and knees. Hands should be placed on the floor slightly in front of your shoulders. Your knees should be placed so that your thighs are at right angles to your torso and to your lower legs. Make sure your back is naturally straight, without straining. Breathe in and let your stomach flop toward the floor. Really let it hang out!

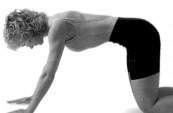

❷ As you breathe out, pull your abdomen up toward the ceiling in a smooth, flowing movement. Don't jerk—the movement should be slow and controlled. Don't arch your back; keep it straight throughout the exercise.

❸ Repeat this ten times, without pausing between repetitions, so it is a fluid, up and down movement. The abdominal muscles are doing all the work. You shouldn't feel any strain in your lower back. Stop immediately and adjust your position if you do.

TAKE CARE

If you have wrist problems, try placing a small rolled-up towel under your hands so that your wrists aren't bent back to such a degree, or just do the other versions of static abs on pages 52–3. Avoid this position if kneeling exacerbates existing knee conditions.

Static Abs

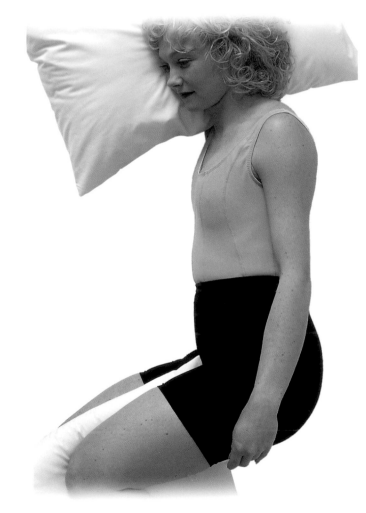

LYING ON YOUR SIDE

❶ Lie on your side in the fetal position with your knees curled up. Place a small pillow between your legs and another one under your head. Your spine should be slightly curved. Adjust your position until you feel comfortable. Breathe in, letting your stomach flop down toward the floor.

2 As you breathe out, pull your stomach upward and back through your spine in an L-shaped movement. Repeat this ten times, then turn onto your other side for ten repetitions that way.

SEMISUPINE

1 Lie on your back with your knees bent and feet slightly apart, in line with your hip joints. Place a small flat cushion between your thighs. Support your head with a small cushion or pillow so that your neck is straight and your shoulders are relaxed into the floor. Place your hands on your abdomen. Breathe into the lower abdomen, letting the air push your hands upward.

2 As you breathe out, pull your abdomen toward the floor. Keep your chest soft and relaxed. Repeat this ten times.

TAKE CARE

If you have a pronounced arch in your lower back, place a pillow under your upper back when you are in the semisupine position. *See the advice on lordosis on pages 19–20.*

Leg Lifts and Slides

These exercises work the muscles to the sides of the lower abdomen, just inside the hip bones. As you start to breathe out, make sure your abdomen is pulled toward the floor before you begin the movement so you don't strain your lower back. Another common mistake is to tense the muscles on the leg that is not moving. Slow down and make the movements smaller until you can feel them working in the right place. Putting your hands on the muscles helps you to double-check.

SINGLE LEG LIFTS

❶ Lie on your back with your knees bent and your weight balanced in the center of your feet. Support your neck with a cushion. Place your hands on your abdomen, as though you are sliding them into an apron pocket. Breathe in.

❷ As you breathe out, pull your navel to the floor and then lift one leg from the ground. Keep your knee bent at the same angle and don't flex your foot as you pull your knee upward. You should feel your lower abdominals working.

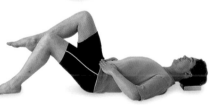

TAKE CARE

If the lift is too much for you when you lie on your back with your knees bent, rest both feet on the edge of a low stool or a pile of books. This will make the lift easier. If you suffer from lordosis (see pages 19–20), you should only do this exercise with your feet raised in this way.

❸ Breathe in. Breathe out as you lower your foot to the floor again in a smooth, controlled movement. Do ten repetitions with each leg, making sure your abdominals do the work.

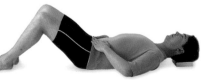

SLIDING ON A CHAIR

❶ Lie on your back with your calves resting on a chair that is the correct height to give you a right angle at the knees and hips. Support your neck with a cushion or a paperback book, then let your shoulders melt into the floor and your lower back fall gently into its natural position; don't try to force your back down to the floor. Breathe in.

❷ As you breathe out, pull your navel to the floor and then slide one heel toward you. Don't let your back arch.

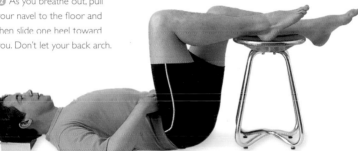

❸ Breathe in. Breathe out while sliding your heel back to the starting position. Repeat ten times with each leg.

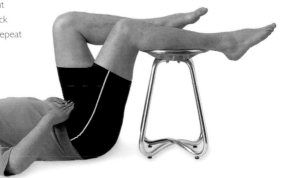

Abdominal Curls

First of all, forget about any previous methods you may have learned for doing sit-ups. The way they are taught in many gyms and exercise classes focuses solely on the rectus abdominis muscle and can place a severe strain on the neck and lower back. Pilates abdominal curls are designed to help you isolate and strengthen all the abdominal muscles without straining anywhere else. Focus hard, putting your thoughts into the muscles you are working, and build up very gradually.

THE BASIC CURL

❶ Lie on your back with your knees bent and the weight balanced in the center of your feet. Hold a small flat cushion loosely between your thighs to keep your pelvis aligned and activate the inner thigh adductors. Clasp your hands behind your head at the base of the skull, keeping your elbows roughly in line with your nose. Imagine there is a tennis ball under your chin, and try to stop it dropping into your chest. Once you have got this position, breathe in.

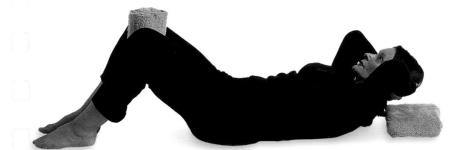

2 As you breathe out, pull your navel to the floor. When you feel the abdominal muscles engaging, lift your head and start to curl forward, letting your ribs move toward your hips. Look straight ahead, between your thighs. Don't pull your head forward with your hands; just support its weight.

3 Don't try to curl too far. When you reach as far as you can go comfortably, without jerking, slowly uncurl back to the starting position, breathing in.

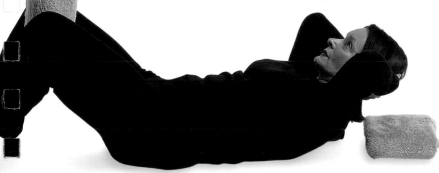

Abdominal Curl Checklist

It's extremely important to make sure that you are doing this movement correctly to avoid injury, so run through the following checklist before doing any repetitions:

● Can you feel any strain on your neck? Are the muscles that run down beneath your ears standing out as you curl forward? If this is the case, try variation 3, described on page 61, where you use a towel to support your head. Always stop exercising immediately if you feel any neck strain.

● Do you feel any strain in your lower back? If so, this means that your abdominal muscles aren't properly engaged. When you start to breathe out, the first 25 percent of the outbreath should be spent pulling your navel to the floor. Don't start the curl until you can feel that the abdominals are engaged. If you suffer from lordosis, make sure that you do this exercise with your feet up (see *variation 2 on page 61*).

● Are you managing to do only a very small curl forward? This is fine. The Pilates abdominal curl should be a small movement, using the muscles correctly. As you become stronger, you will be able to curve farther forward. Don't ever try to emulate the fitness-freaks you see in gyms who are virtually touching their foreheads to their knees, while their veins bulge with the effort!

● If your abdomen "pops out" or the muscles bunch up as you're curling, you're going too far. Your ribs shouldn't lift above the height of your hips. Think instead about your rib cage softening as you curl forward.

● Can you feel a strain in your inner thighs? This probably means you are grasping the cushion between them. Try variation 2 on page 61, where you have your feet up.

Once you're confident that you are doing the curl correctly, just working the abdominals, do ten repetitions. Try variation 1 on page 60 as well.

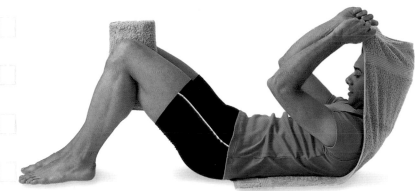

Using a towel
Do you have a neck problem or feel a strain on your neck during ab curl exercises?
If so, try the ab curl variation with a towel on page 61.

Ab Curl Variations

If you have had trouble working the right muscles during the basic curl on page 56, it's definitely worth trying one or more of these alternative versions to set you on the right track. Choose the one that works best for you and do your curls this way for a few weeks until your abdominals are stronger.

VARIATION 1—WALKING FINGERS

This is a variation of the basic curl, which can help to ensure you are moving in the correct direction. However, your hands aren't providing any support for the weight of the head, so make sure you aren't straining your neck.

❶ Lie on your back with your knees bent and your feet on the ground. Hold a flat cushion between your knees. Rest your hands lightly on your thighs. Breathe in.

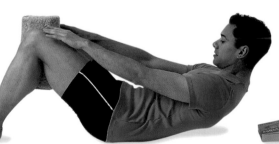

❷ As you breathe out, engage the abdominal muscles first, bring your head forward, look at your thighs, then start walking your fingers up your thighs toward your knees.

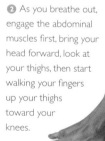

❸ When you reach the top of the curl, stop and breathe in. Breathe out again as you uncurl slowly back to the floor.

NOTE

If you are still having trouble with your ab curls after trying these variations, do the alternative reverse curl on page 63.

VARIATION 2—WITH FEET UP

*This variation helps to support the lower back and stops you
from engaging your thigh muscles, so it is much easier to
isolate the abdominal muscles.*

❶ Find a stool or arrange a pile
of cushions at a height so that when
you place your legs on top of them,
your knees and hips are at right
angles; however, it shouldn't be so
high that your hips are lifting off the
floor. Hold a flat cushion between your
knees. Keep your knees in line with your hip joints and
flex your feet very slightly. Put your hands behind your
head, clasping them lightly. Breathe in.

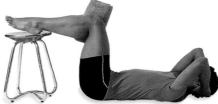

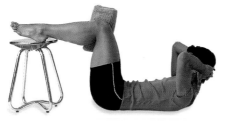

❷ As you breathe out, pull your
navel to the floor and then curl
forward. At the top of the curl,
breathe in, then uncurl again while
breathing out. Make sure your
abdominals are doing the work
and that you are not pressing
down on your heels.

VARIATION 3—WITH TOWEL

*This method is helpful for people who have any kind of
neck problems or bunched-up muscles in their shoulders.*

❶ Place a small towel under your upper back so that it
extends about 2 in. (5 cm) above the top of your head
when you are lying down. Hold the top corners
of the towel lightly between your finger and
thumb, keeping your lower arms parallel. Get
into position for the curl, with your knees
bent and feet on the floor. Breathe in.

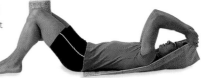

❷ Breathe out and sink your navel to the floor.
Lift your head slightly and then pull the towel
so it is supporting your head as you curl
forward, moving your elbows toward your hip
joints. At the top of the curl, breathe in, then
uncurl again while breathing out. After doing
this for a few weeks, you may find you
don't need the towel any more.

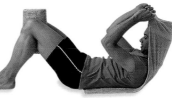

Reverse Curls

These work a slightly different area of the abdominals. Choose a solid piece of furniture that is not going to move during the exercise. While the basic reverse curl is an advanced exercise and should not be attempted until you can do the basic curl confidently, the alternative reverse curl is good for people with weak abdominals; unlike the other curls, you've got gravity on your side.

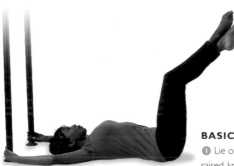

BASIC REVERSE CURL

❶ Lie on your back with your legs raised, knees slightly bent and shoulder-width apart, and your ankles crossed. Extend your hands behind your head and hold onto a sturdy piece of furniture. Breathe in.

❷ Breathe out, sink your navel to the floor, and pull your knees toward your chest. Your pelvis will curl off the floor a little. Breathe in, then breathe out as you move your knees back to the starting position.

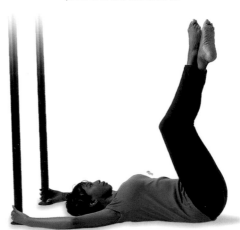

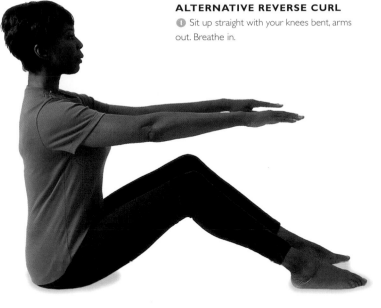

ALTERNATIVE REVERSE CURL

1 Sit up straight with your knees bent, arms out. Breathe in.

2 As you breathe out, engage the abdominals and then roll your upper body down to the floor, using your stomach muscles to control the curl back. Use your arms to push back up to the starting position. Repeat ten times.

TAKE CARE

Don't try reverse curls if you suffer from back or hip problems, and stop immediately if you feel any pain in your lower back.

Cross-fiber Ab Curls

These will work the abdominal muscles at the sides. Make sure that your hips, legs, and lower-to-middle spine don't move during the exercise. Don't rush; keep it very slow. If you use a towel to support your neck during the basic ab curls, you should do the same here. You will have to hold the towel with both hands, rather than stretching one arm across your body. You can also do cross-fiber ab curls with your feet up on a box if you have lower back problems.

① Adopt the same semisupine starting position as for the basic ab curl. Put your left hand behind your head and cross your right arm across your torso, aiming your right hand toward the outside of your left knee. The hand should be in the shape of a loose fist. Breathe in.

2 Breathe out, engage your abdominals, lift your head slightly, and stretch across to the left side, as if you are trying to fold your right shoulder to your left hip. It should be a smooth movement in the same direction; don't lift up first and then turn sideways.

3 When you reach the extent of your curl, pause, then breathe in as you curl back down to the starting position. Repeat ten times, then do the same curl in the other direction, with your right hand behind your head and your left hand stretched across your body, curling your left shoulder toward your right hip.

Small Hip Rolls

With the small hip rolls, you will feel a stretch in your lower abdominal muscles, just above the bladder. Don't try to move your knees too far; this is a very tiny movement. The larger hip rolls on pages 68–69 give a wonderful stretch diagonally across the abdomen from hip to ribs. In this one, stretch as far as you can.

❶ Lie on your back with your knees bent and feet together. Arrange cushions under your head and/or upper back. Place your hands on your abdominals just above your hip bones. Breathe in.

REPETITIONS

If you can't manage the number of repetitions an exercise asks you to do, don't worry about it. Just do as many as you can and build up gradually. If you are exhausted after five, just do four. You'll be amazed how quickly your strength builds and you find you can manage more. On the other hand, if a stretch is easy, it probably means you don't need to stretch that area, so move onto another area. Don't do more repetitions than you are asked to. Some of the exercises are progressive and you can move onto the next stage.

2 As you breathe out, engage the abdominals and move your knees to the right, keeping your hips on the floor. Use your left hand to help pull the abdominals in the opposite direction; this will help to keep the hips in place. Breathe in.

3 Breathe out and pull your navel to the floor before moving your knees across to the left, using your right hand to pull your abdominals to the right. Repeat this ten times.

Larger Hip Rolls

Hip rolls feel great and are a good way to loosen up during a session. Just make sure you keep your abdominals engaged, so that they do the work of bringing your knees up from the side, to the center, and across, or you could strain your lower back.

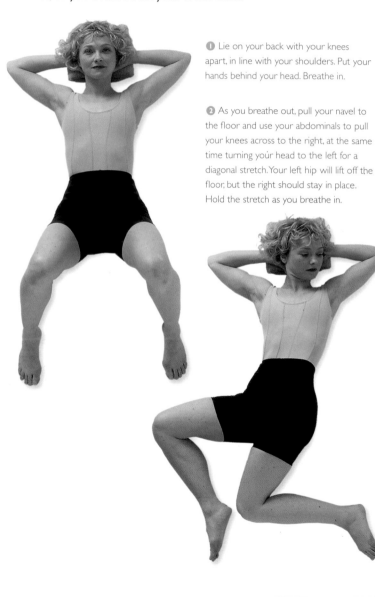

❶ Lie on your back with your knees apart, in line with your shoulders. Put your hands behind your head. Breathe in.

❷ As you breathe out, pull your navel to the floor and use your abdominals to pull your knees across to the right, at the same time turning your head to the left for a diagonal stretch. Your left hip will lift off the floor, but the right should stay in place. Hold the stretch as you breathe in.

③ Breathe out, engage your abdominals, and pull your knees up to the center and to the left, turning your head to the right. Repeat ten times.

VARIATION—WITH EXERCISE BALL

If you have an exercise ball, try resting your legs on it to do hip rolls. Exercise balls are widely available by mail order and from many stores.

Single Leg Stretches

You need to keep your abdominal muscles pulled in throughout this exercise while breathing into your lungs, so don't attempt it until you are confident that your abdomen is strong enough. If you can manage ten basic ab curls, you should be fine. If you feel a strain in your neck, you could support your neck and shoulders with a pillow folded in half.

❶ Lie on your back with your knees bent into your chest, shoulder-width apart. Hold your knees loosely with your hands, elbows pointing outward. Breathe in.

❷ As you breathe out, engage your abdominals and curl your head and upper torso forward.

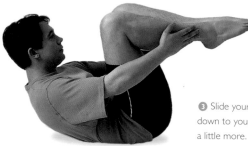

❸ Slide your hands from your knees down to your ankles, curling forward a little more. Breathe in.

④ As you breathe out, stretch out your right leg and take hold of your left knee with your right hand. Don't try to lift your right foot too high; approximately in line with your shoulder is fine. Maintain the curve of your upper torso, keeping your elbows up and shoulders down.

TAKE CARE

This is an advanced exercise and is not suitable for people with lower back pain or hip problems.

⑤ As you breathe in, change legs. Take hold of your right knee with your left hand and your right ankle with your right hand. Don't use your hands to pull the legs; they should merely be guiding them. Do eight repetitions on each side.

VARIATION—WITHOUT HOLDING

In this variation, instead of holding the knees and ankles, you stretch your arms out at an angle of approximately 45° to your torso. Hold this position and keep your abdominals engaged as you repeat steps 4 and 5 of the single leg stretches at least 5 times. This is much harder!

The Cobra

This is a useful exercise for stretching out the abdominal muscles after you have been working them and also helps to strengthen the muscles of the lower back. Do the movements very gently to begin with, and don't try this if you have lower back problems—do the alternative stretch instead.

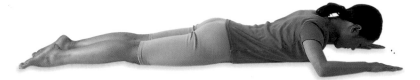

❶ Lie face down with your forehead resting on the floor or a small flat cushion (this is known as the "prone" position). Your arms should be bent by the sides of your head with the palms facing downward. Breathe in.

❷ As you breathe out, lift your head, neck, and shoulders as far as you can from the floor, and hold for a few seconds. Don't push with your arms; use the muscles of your torso to lift you. Feel the stretch in your stomach and your shoulderblades drawing down toward your pelvis. Breathe in.

❸ Breathe out and lower your upper body gradually back to the starting position.

NOTE

You may not be able to stretch back as far as our model on your first attempts. Don't force it. Go as far as you can manage comfortably and then breathe in, holding the position, before you curl down again. Gradually, you will find you are able to stretch a little farther each time.

ALTERNATIVE STRETCH

If you have lower back pain and can't manage the Cobra, try this instead. Place your hands in the small of your back, breathe out, and engage your abdominals, then draw your upper torso backward. Don't try to go too far. You should feel the stretch in your abdomen.

VARIATION—WITH STRAIGHT ARMS

1 Lie face down with your arms stretched straight forward on either side of your head. Rest your forehead on a small cushion, if you wish. Breathe in.

2 As you breathe out, draw your shoulderblades down your back, lift your head and breastbone, and slide your arms along the floor towards you. Hold this position for a few seconds, keeping your arms straight.

3 Breathe in as you slowly return to the starting position.

Questions & Answers

Q Can abdominal muscles ever be too strong?

A Yes, they can. Abdominal strength shouldn't be out of proportion, otherwise the muscles can restrict movements, such as bending and stretching, and put strain on the back. Weight lifters could be at risk of overstrengthening this area.

Q I'm still having trouble with the ab curls. Sometimes I manage one or two that feel right, but I can't sustain it.

A Don't despair. Keep practicing the static abs, cross-fiber ab curls, and the alternative reverse curl on page 63. After a couple of weeks of focusing on these, go back and try your basic ab curls again, and you should see a difference.

Q I've given birth to four children, and I don't think there's a functioning muscle left in my belly. Is there anything I can do to get the strength back?

A Your muscle tone will come back if you keep exercising the area gently. You should concentrate on the abdominal exercises in this section and also make sure you are doing the pelvic floor exercises on page 78 every day. See your physician if you don't feel you are making any progress after six weeks of regular exercise.

Q My husband does abdominal curls very quickly, with lots of repetitions at a time. Why is the Pilates version so much slower?

A We do ab curls slowly to use the breath properly and to make sure the back muscles are disengaged as much as possible. If you do them too quickly, your abdomen will pop out and you won't be using the correct muscles any more.

Q I don't understand how strong abdominals can relieve digestive problems. How does it work?

A When your abdominals hold the organs in the correct positions, the squeezing movements of the digestive system, which pass waste materials downward, work more efficiently. There is also evidence that some digestive disorders are caused by stress-related cramping of the gut, so any activities that relieve stress can be helpful.

Q Which are the best Pilates exercises for getting rid of "love handles"?

A Cross-fiber ab curls are great for this area, and so is the double leg lift, described on page 165. If you are focusing on this area in a Pilates session, do some side stretches afterward (see pages 132–33).

Q Should I always do a stretch after abdominal exercises?

A It's best to do a small stretch, even if it's just lying on the floor with your arms extended above your head, then stretching your fingers and heels away from each other.

Q I get a stitch in my side with the cross-fiber ab curls. What does this mean and how can I avoid it?

A A stitch is an involuntary contraction of a muscle. Stop and rub the area when this happens. You could try a stretch to relieve it, or a small hip roll, or just relax for a while and try again.

The Pelvic Area

In the posture section, we discussed the importance of the pelvis being correctly aligned. If you've never had any problems in this area, you probably take it for granted that your pelvis is fine, but it may not be if any of the following apply to you:

- you have poor posture and/or weak stomach muscles;
- you are prone to sitting with your legs crossed;
- you are an athlete;
- you are pregnant (read pages 190–95 before trying the exercises in this section);
- you lift heavy weights at work or at home, or do weight training;
- you often wear unsuitable shoes, such as high heels.

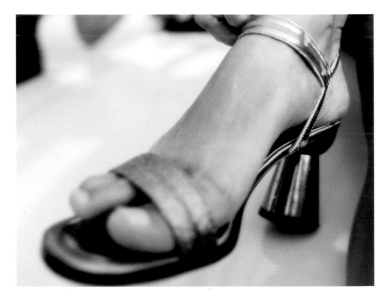

High heels
Shoes with high heels tilt the pelvis forward, so you are forced to lean backward
to keep your balance, creating an arch in your lower back.

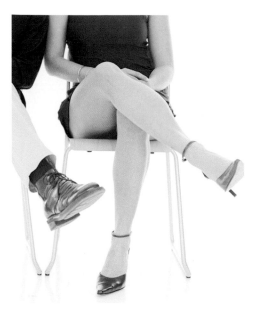

Crossed legs
If you are more comfortable crossing your legs one way than the other, it is because the muscles that support your pelvis have contracted to support you this way after years of habitual leg-crossing.

The quadriceps, running down the front of the thighs from the hips to the knees, are the largest muscle group in the body. From when we are babies, they do a lot of work without any conscious effort on our part: kicking, crawling, walking, running, jumping, sitting down, standing up. If the quads are too strong, they are not effectively counterbalanced by the hamstrings, and can cause the pelvis to tilt forward. In this section, we will look at strengthening the muscles that support the pelvis in its correct position, all of which are vital to core stability. These are the gluteus maximus, running across the buttocks; the inner thigh muscles, running from the knee to the pelvis; and the hamstrings, which bend the legs and let them swing backward and forward from the hips. Don't forget the postural tips for correct alignment of the pelvis: keep your hips square and level; when standing, your feet should be directly under your hips; always bend forward from the hip joint rather than the upper back or waist.

Pelvic Floor Muscles

The pelvic floor muscles control the sphincter muscles at the openings of the anus, vagina (in women), and urethra. If these muscles are not exercised, they will weaken and the results can be involuntary leakage of urine at inappropriate moments, prolapse of the uterus (in women), and even loss of bowel control. Here's what to do:

● Sit in a chair with your knees slightly apart and feet on the floor. It can help to identify the pelvic floor muscles if you lean forward slightly from the hips. Tighten and pull up the muscle around your anus, hold it for five seconds if you can, then relax. Repeat five times, then tighten the muscle quickly five times, relaxing immediately after each squeeze.

● Concentrate on the vaginal muscles: draw them up and in, and hold for five seconds. If you are unsure whether you are using the correct muscles, try inserting two fingers into your vagina. You should feel a gentle squeeze. Repeat this five times, holding the squeeze for five seconds, then five times quickly, relaxing after each squeeze.

● At least once a day, do the "stop test" when urinating. Stop your urine in midflow, hold for five seconds, then release it again.

Do the first two steps—five slow and five fast—at least ten times a day. As the muscles get stronger, you will find you can manage more repetitions and hold them for longer.

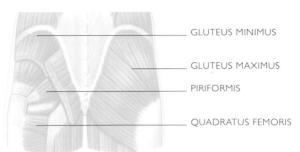

GLUTEUS MINIMUS

GLUTEUS MAXIMUS

PIRIFORMIS

QUADRATUS FEMORIS

Buttock muscles

These help to support the pelvis
in its correct alignment.

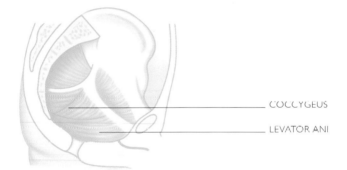

COCCYGEUS

LEVATOR ANI

Pelvic floor muscles

Men can find their pelvic floor is
weakened after prostate treatments.

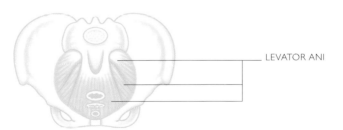

LEVATOR ANI

Pelvic floor muscles

It's vitally important that women do their
pelvic floor exercises regularly during and
after pregnancy.

Glute Squeezes

Strong gluteus maximus muscles are crucial for maintaining core stability and they are also very important for walking. If older people are prone to tripping, it is often because they have weak glutes and are having to tilt their pelvis in order to lift each leg clear of the ground when walking. When you start these exercises, you may find that the muscles are stronger on one side than the other. If that's the case, try engaging the weak side first, then the stronger side, and you'll find that they even up in strength fairly quickly. If you have trouble locating the correct muscles when lying down, start with standing glute squeezes (*see pages 82–83*).

LYING GLUTE SQUEEZE

❶ Lie on your front with a pillow under your abdomen to support the lower back and prevent it from arching. Roll up a small towel (*see note opposite*) and place it between your upper thighs to help focus the movement. If you have tension in your shoulders, you can place a pillow underneath them, or roll up two small towels and place one under each shoulder. Experiment until you are comfortable and your upper back is relaxed. Bend your elbows and rest your forehead on your hands. Breathe in.

USING A ROLLED-UP TOWEL

A useful tool for some exercises is a hand towel rolled up tightly and secured, if necessary, with elastic bands at both ends. Make sure it is not more than 2 in. (5 cm) in diameter. This can be used between the knees to maintain pelvic alignment in the semisupine position, or placed underneath the lower ribs to help relax the shoulders and open the chest when doing upper torso exercises. It can also be used to protect the knees when doing the hamstring curls on pages 84–85 (see *caution box*).

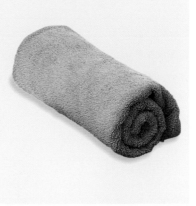

7 As you breathe out, imagine you are squeezing your sitting bones together. The bones won't actually move, but this helps to pull the glutes in the right way. Hold the squeeze for four seconds. Make sure your legs don't rotate; they should stay completely still. Relax and repeat ten times.

Standing Glute Squeeze

Many people find it easier to locate the glute muscles in a standing position. Watch that your thighs don't turn inward when you squeeze your glutes. Feel the difference when you squeeze with your feet parallel, and then turned out at an angle.

1 Stand straight, leaning your hands against a wall or holding onto a door for support. Your feet should be parallel and slightly apart, placed directly under your hips. Breathe in and squeeze your glutes as you breathe out, holding for four seconds. You will feel a gentle stretching in your lower back and a lifting of the stomach muscles as they automatically engage during this movement. Keep your weight firmly balanced on your feet throughout the squeeze; don't let your legs rotate outward.

② From the same starting position, breathe in and squeeze your buttocks together, holding for four seconds. As you breathe out, rise up onto your toes, holding onto the door or leaning against the wall for support. This movement will also work your calf muscles.

❸ Stand with your legs rotated slightly outward so there is an angle of roughly 60° between your feet. Hold onto the door or lean your hands on a wall. Breathe in and squeeze your glutes as you breathe out, holding for four seconds. This exercises the glutes slightly farther out than when you stand with feet parallel.

Hamstring Curls

It's very important to make sure your legs are completely parallel when doing hamstring curls, but it's difficult to see for yourself. Many people's legs lie at slightly different degrees of rotation without them being aware of it. Lie on your front and ask a friend to stand at your feet and adjust your legs until they are perfectly straight. It may feel "wrong" at first, but try to memorize this position and adopt it every time you do hamstring curls. Let your friend watch as you do the exercise, to make sure you are keeping your foot in line with your hip as you bend your leg, and not letting it stray out to the side.

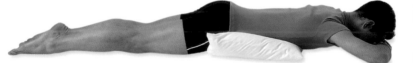

❶ Lie on your front, using cushions or small towels to support your lower back and shoulders, as you did for the lying glute squeezes. Rest your forehead on your hands. Don't hold a towel between your legs this time, but make sure they are straight and parallel. Breathe in.

TAKE CARE

If you have knee problems, try placing a rolled towel underneath your thighs, just above the knees, so your kneecaps are not pressing on the floor. If these exercises still feel uncomfortable around your knees, don't do them until your leg muscles are stronger.

❷ As you breathe out, slowly bend one leg up until your knee is at an angle of 90°, keeping your foot soft and in line with your hip.

❸ Breathe in as you lower your foot to the ground again. Do ten repetitions with each leg, aiming to make the movements smooth and flowing. Keep them slow and make sure you can feel the muscles at the back of your thighs working.

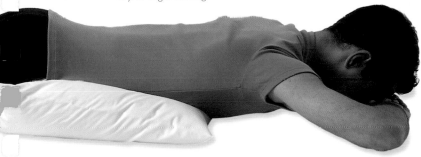

Hamstring Curl Variations

Aim to do your hamstring curls in a smooth, flowing rhythm, without jerking. If you find this difficult, make the movement smaller. Do not try these variations until you are able to do ten smooth repetitions of the basic hamstring curl with each leg.

VARIATION I—ARM ABOVE HEAD

On the side you are doing the hamstring curl, stretch your arm straight out above your head with your fingers extended. This will help you to visualize the straight line your leg should be moving in.

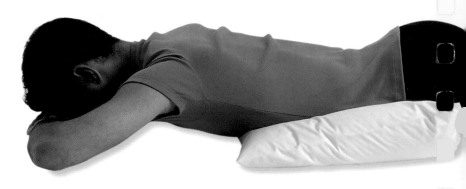

VARIATION 2—OPENING THE HIP

*When your knee is bent at 90°, let your leg drop
open to the side. You should feel a sensation of
the hip opening out. Straighten up again before
you lower your leg to the ground.*

VARIATION 3—LIFTING THE KNEE

*When your knee is bent at 90°, lift it slightly off the
ground. Bring it down again before you lower your foot
to the floor. This is an advanced variation and you
shouldn't try it until your core stability is strong, or
you could risk straining your lower back.*

Pelvic Tilts

These exercises are progressive. Make sure you master stage 1 before you try stage 2, and that you can do stage 2 confidently before going onto stage 3, which requires more strength in your abdominal muscles. Perform the movements very slowly so that you curl up gradually, bit by bit, and come down again in a controlled manner using the muscles of your torso and feeling the stretch in your back.

NOTE

Women suffering from period pains may find that small pelvic tilts help to relieve them. Sink your navel to the floor and curl up your tailbone slightly to ease the discomfort.

STAGE 1

① Lie on your back with your knees bent, feet on the floor, and directly in line with your hips. Place a small flat cushion or rolled-up towel between your thighs to maintain the alignment of the pelvis. Support your head with a small cushion so your neck is straight and rest your arms by your sides. Relax your shoulders into the floor. Breathe in.

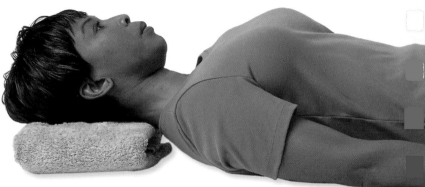

② As you breathe out, sink your navel to the floor and then pull up your pelvic floor and curl your tailbone upward, feeling the pelvis tilt. Imagine you are curling your tailbone between your legs toward your navel. Keep your shoulders and upper back soft and relaxed into the floor. Make sure you aren't squeezing the cushion between your thighs; just hold it in position. Breathe in.

③ Breathe out and slowly curl down to the starting position again. Repeat this pelvic tilt ten times.

Pelvic Tilts

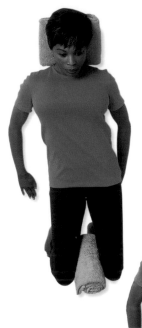

STAGE 2

① Adopt the same starting position as for stage 1, but this time you will curl up a little farther. Breathe out, drop your navel to the floor, pull up your pelvic floor, and then curl upward until your waist is just lifted off the floor. Breathe in.

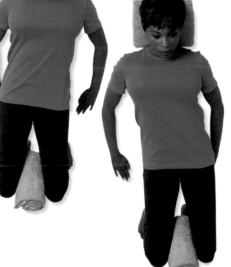

② Breathe out and swing your hips to one side and then the other, thinking of them forming an arc shape in the air. Your knees shouldn't move and your shoulders and upper back should stay relaxed into the floor. Repeat the swing a few times, then return your hips to the center and breathe in.

③ Breathe out and curl gradually back down to the floor. Repeat ten times.

> ### TAKE CARE
> If you have neck or shoulder problems, stage 3 of this exercise may be uncomfortable for you. Just concentrate on perfecting stages 1 and 2.

STAGE 3

① Adopt the same starting position and this time let your curl take you right up until you are resting on your shoulderblades. Look down toward your knees to keep your neck lengthened. Keep your abdominals engaged throughout.

② Breathe in and raise your hands up to the ceiling, then stretch them onto the floor behind you.

③ Leaving your arms behind you, breathe out as you curl down slowly: first the ribs, then the waist, lower spine, and finally the pelvis. Feel the stretch in your arms and torso.

④ Breathe in and return your arms to your sides, either back over your head or in a large circular movement around the floor. Repeat stage 3 ten times.

Adductor Cushion Squeeze

This is a useful exercise for isolating and strengthening the inner thigh adductor muscles and is a good preparation for the other inner thigh exercises on pages 162–63 and 166–67. You may feel your glutes engaging as well, but concentrate on the inner thighs and make sure that you can feel them working.

● Lie on your back with your knees bent and your feet slightly apart. Place a small cushion or a rolled-up towel between your knees. Breathe out and pull the inner thighs together, gently squeezing but not gripping the cushion or towel. Hold for four counts before releasing.

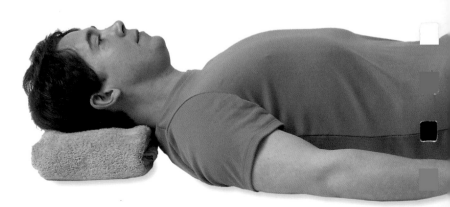

VARIATION—WITH AB CURL

Follow the directions for the cushion squeeze, left, then sink your navel to the floor and add a small abdominal curl with *your hands behind your head (see page 56) or by walking your fingers up your thighs (see page 60).*

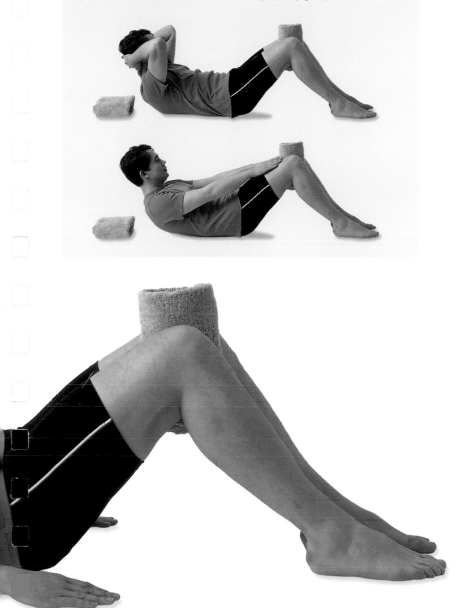

The Shake

This is a lovely exercise for releasing the lower back while stretching the abdominal muscles, so it's a good one to do after a session when you've been working on the abdomen and pelvis.

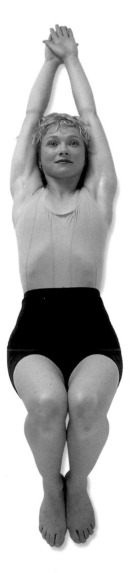

❶ Lie on your back with your knees bent and your knees and feet together. Place your arms straight behind your head, one hand on top of the other, resting them on a pillow if necessary to avoid any strain in the shoulder joints.

TAKE CARE

Go easy on the Shake if you are prone to lower back pain.

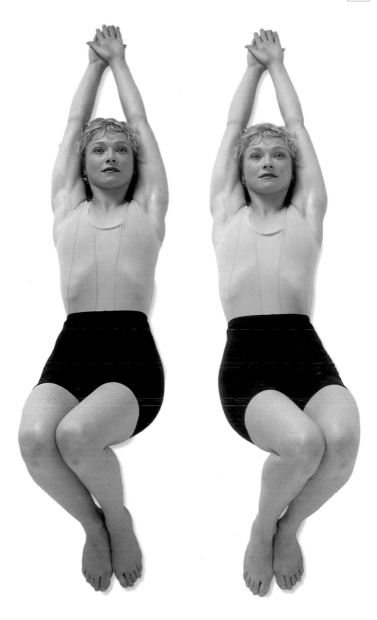

❷ Gently rock your knees from side to side, like a metronome, as you stretch your arms. Keep your feet flat on the floor. Let your hips move naturally. Your stomach muscles should be working gently and you should breathe normally.

Questions & Answers

Q I get cramps in my hamstrings when doing pelvic tilts. What am I doing wrong?

A You are gripping your thighs and pressing into your feet, instead of using the pelvic and abdominal muscles to tilt. Try putting your legs up on a chair. Alternatively, you can buy an exercise ball to rest your legs on.

Q Which Pilates exercises are good for a flabby, out-of-shape bottom?

A The most effective exercises are the glute squeezes. Do them everywhere: standing at the kitchen sink or in the checkout line at the supermarket. Hamstring curls are also good, as is an exercise called the Shell on pages 168–69.

Q I can't do pelvic floor exercises and breathe at the same time. Does this mean I'm doing them incorrectly?

A It is possible to do pelvic floor exercises without breathing, but they will be much more effective combined with correct breathing. You must be trying to squeeze so hard that all your upper torso muscles are tensing. Try a smaller squeeze next time.

Q If I lie on my front, it feels "wrong" when I straighten my legs in line with my hips. Can I work with my legs slightly to one side?

A No; this is a bad postural habit that you must try to correct. It feels odd because it's not what you've become used to, but you should persevere and work with your body straight.

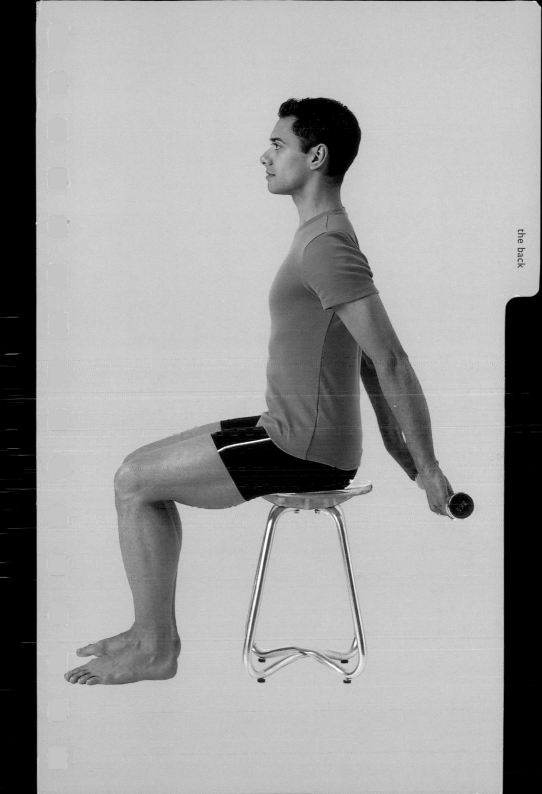

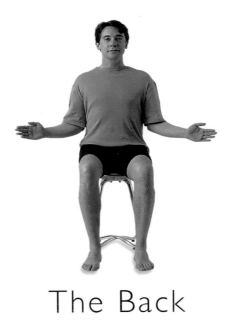

The Back

The back is one of the most vulnerable areas of the body.
Almost everyone will suffer from back pain at some time in their
lives and it is one of the biggest causes of lost work hours in the
Western world. Those who have to lift and carry heavy loads on
a regular basis are particularly vulnerable, and so are people who
have a desk job that entails long hours sitting in the same position.
Pregnancy can cause back problems (see *pages 190–95*) and so
can being overweight, because the back has more weight to support
and the abdominals tend to be weaker. Pilates can help to prevent
back pain, by strengthening the back muscles while the spine is
held in the correct alignment. It can also alleviate existing back
weaknesses, but you should check with your specialist first if
you suffer from chronic back pain.

The Back

Although injuries and some diseases can cause back pain, much of it derives from bad posture. When the postural alignment is consistently wrong, the muscles contract and put strain on the spinal joints. Acute back pain, or "putting your back out," is usually the result of one "final straw" after years of incorrect posture have weakened the muscles, but even strong, fit people can damage their backs if they lift something awkwardly. Never twist around when lifting. If you are sitting in the driver's seat of your car and need to get a bag from the back seat, don't be tempted to turn around and haul it over; get out of the car first and take the bag out of the back door.

Core stability is the key to supporting the back and the rest of the body correctly, so it's crucial to work on the abdominals, pelvis, glutes, and hamstrings to help protect yourself from back pain. In this chapter, we will look at the main muscle groups that are used to move and support the back: the latissimus dorsi muscles, which help to stabilize

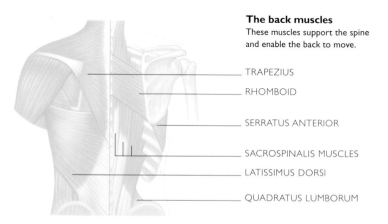

The back muscles
These muscles support the spine and enable the back to move.

TRAPEZIUS

RHOMBOID

SERRATUS ANTERIOR

SACROSPINALIS MUSCLES

LATISSIMUS DORSI

QUADRATUS LUMBORUM

the upper torso; the serratus anterior, which draws the shoulderblades forward against the ribs; the rhomboids, which pull the shoulderblades around the spine; the sacrospinalis muscles, which enable us to bend backward and twist sideways; the

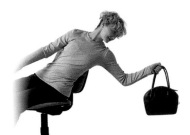

Twisting and lifting
The strain of lifting when you're in an unstable position can be enough to "put your back out."

quadratus lumborum, used for side bending; and the large trapezius muscle, whose lower part helps to maintain the spine in a straight line while the upper and middle parts adduct and lift the shoulderblades.

Back problems

If you suffer from back pain, it is important to seek medical advice and get an accurate diagnosis before attempting any exercise. The causes could range from ligament strain, muscle tear, or damage to a spinal joint, through to disk prolapse or osteoarthritis, and different treatments would be recommended for each. There are also certain types of exercise that should be avoided in each case, so as not to exacerbate the problem. If you are prone to lower back pain, you should place a cushion under your stomach to support the arch of the spine during any exercises that are performed lying on your front. Always do abdominal curls and pelvic tilts with your feet up. Watch out for the caution boxes beside some exercises in this book, which will tell you when to take it easy. In all cases of back pain, listen to your body and judge for yourself. Stop immediately if you feel any strain.

The Arrow

Do not try to lift too far off the floor in this exercise, and never bend your head backward. Keep your torso long and contract your back muscles, elongating the front and pulling your shoulderblades down. You should almost feel as though your head is being pulled away from your body.

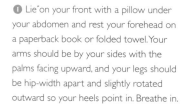

❶ Lie on your front with a pillow under your abdomen and rest your forehead on a paperback book or folded towel. Your arms should be by your sides with the palms facing upward, and your legs should be hip-width apart and slightly rotated outward so your heels point in. Breathe in.

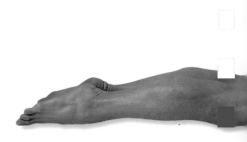

TAKE CARE

Try these exercises very carefully if you suffer from lower back pain. Make sure your abdominals are engaged and stop if you feel any twinges.

❷ Breathe out, engage your abdominals, and let your palms float up until they are roughly level with your hips. Gently pull down your shoulderblades toward your buttocks and lift your head and breastbone away from the floor without bending your head back. As you lift, you should feel the muscles below your shoulderblades working.

❸ Breathe in to return to starting position. Repeat ten times.

The Star

Like the Arrow, this exercise strengthens your lower torso, but this time the lift is diagonal. The movements should be smooth and flowing, almost as if you are swimming. You should feel a nice easy stretch through the whole torso from your fingers to your toes, but make sure you keep your shoulders relaxed throughout.

❶ Lie on your front as you did for step 1 of the Arrow, but this time your arms should be extended on the floor above your head, shoulder-width apart, and your palms resting lightly on the floor. Breathe in.

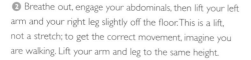

❷ Breathe out, engage your abdominals, then lift your left arm and your right leg slightly off the floor. This is a lift, not a stretch; to get the correct movement, imagine you are walking. Lift your arm and leg to the same height.

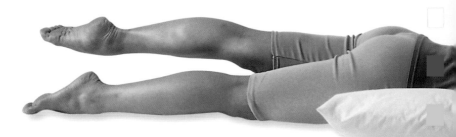

TAKE CARE

If this lift causes discomfort in your lower back, leave it for a while and continue with the Arrow instead.

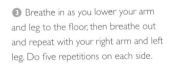

❸ Breathe in as you lower your arm and leg to the floor, then breathe out and repeat with your right arm and left leg. Do five repetitions on each side.

The Cat

The whole length of the spine is stretched in this exercise, and it is particularly good for pregnant women and anyone who suffers from lower back pain, although they should omit step 3. Make your repetitions smooth and flowing, without pausing between them.

❶ Kneel on all fours with your hands shoulder-width apart and your knees hip-width apart. Hold your head so that the spine is naturally straight and your lower back is slightly curved.

TAKE CARE

If you have wrist problems, such as carpal tunnel syndrome, you might find it uncomfortable to extend your wrists backward in this position. Roll up a small towel and hold it in your hands, level with your shoulders. Don't lock your elbows or lean into your arms as you perform the movements. Don't do step 3 if you have lordosis or any kind of lower back pain.

2 Breathe in and slowly round your back upward while letting your head drop down so you are looking at your knees. You should feel the stretch right through the length of your back. Keep the movement smooth and flowing.

3 Breathe out and engage your abdominals, then scoop your back down into a curve so that your head and bottom lift upward. Breathe in to return to the starting point. Repeat ten times.

The Dog

This exercise is great for strengthening the lower back while working the lower abdominals, but don't try it until you have mastered the Cat, because it requires a lot more strength and balance. Do the movements very slowly and keep your abdominals engaged throughout.

● Kneel on all fours, with your knees hip-width apart, your back naturally flat, and your neck straight. Breathe in.

❷ Breathe out, engage your abdominal muscles, and extend your right arm and left leg, stretching them out so they are parallel to the floor. Don't let your back arch. If you have trouble keeping your balance like this, try extending one arm in front, then a leg, and when you feel more comfortable, put both movements together.

VARIATION—CURLING THE ELBOWS

This is the same as the Dog, but more advanced again. It will be hard to keep your balance unless your core stability muscles are strong enough.

❶ The starting position is the same as for step 1 of the Dog. Engage your abdominals and extend your right arm and left leg as for step 2. Breathing in, curl your right elbow and your left knee into the center underneath your torso, gently arching your back upward and letting your head drop forward. Stretch back out again, breathing out.

❷ Repeat with your left arm and right leg. Build up to four repetitions on each diagonal, making sure that you hold your abdominals throughout the movements. You should feel a good stretch in your buttocks and lower back.

TAKE CARE

If you feel tension in your neck and shoulders, check that your weight is evenly balanced between the leg and arm which remain on the ground and that your back is straight. If you suffer from neck problems, you may not be able to do this exercise until your core stability muscles are stronger. The Dog is good for people with lower back pain, if they can manage it. If you have trouble, try it while lying on an exercise ball or across a stool.

❸ Breathe in as you return to the starting position, then repeat step 2 with the left arm and right leg. Do five repetitions on each diagonal.

Sitting Lats

The latissimus dorsi muscles help to control arm movements and are important for stabilizing the upper torso. When they are weak, people tend to compensate by using the shoulder muscles instead, causing strain in the neck and upper back. There are several more exercises to strengthen them in the next lesson.

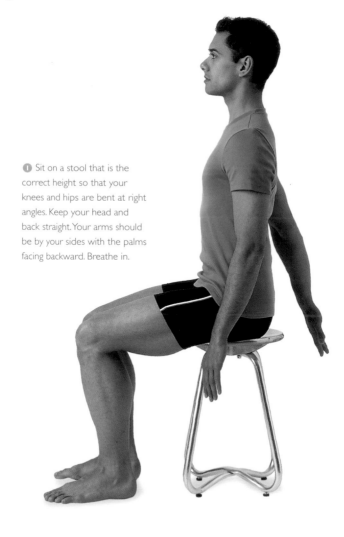

❶ Sit on a stool that is the correct height so that your knees and hips are bent at right angles. Keep your head and back straight. Your arms should be by your sides with the palms facing backward. Breathe in.

TAKE CARE

If you feel any strain in your neck and shoulders, you are doing this incorrectly. Try again, imagining that your arms are light and floating and visualizing your back muscles doing the work. Concentrate on sliding your shoulderblades down so the lats engage. If you still have difficulty feeling the lats working, try variation 2, described on page 111.

❷ As you breathe out, engage your abdominals, then push one palm backward against the air, keeping your shoulders down. Imagine a triangle on your chest, running between your shoulders, with the point at your diaphragm, and try to feel this triangle opening outward as you push back.

❸ Breathe in and return to the starting position. Repeat five times on each side, then five times with both arms together. Don't let your shoulders curl forward.

Sitting Lats Variations

VARIATION 1—WITH WEIGHTS

Once you can perform sitting lats confidently, try doing them while holding some kind of weight in each hand. You may have hand weights at home, but if not, cans of beans will do. Breathe in and, as you breathe out, pull your arms back as in steps 2 and 3 of sitting lats.

ROTATION

Some people who otherwise consider themselves fit have trouble rotating sideways as required in the Sitting Lats Variation with a Belt. There are several exercises in this section to help make the thoracic spine more mobile. Try Cossack Arms (see pages 122–23) and do some Side Stretches (see pages 132–33).

VARIATION 2—WITH A BELT

You'll need some kind of elasticated belt for this, or an old pair of panty hose. Place your chair close to something you can loop the belt around, such as a banister or door handle.

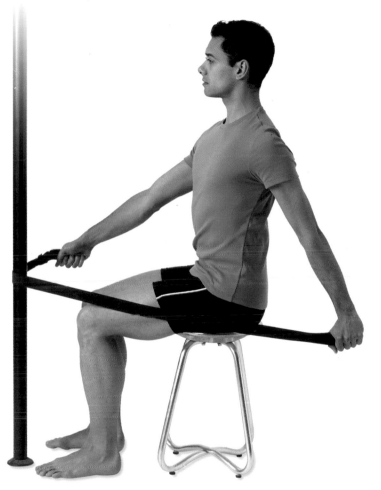

❶ Sit in the starting position for sitting lats with an end of the belt in each hand, so that it is pulled taut when your arms are by your sides. Breathe in.

❷ Breathe out, engage your abdominals, then pull the belt backward with your left arm, so that the right arm is pulled forward naturally. Breathe in.

❸ Breathe out, engage your abdominals, and pull the belt backward with your right arm. Don't consciously move the left arm; just let the right arm pull it forward. Turn your upper body to the right. Repeat five times in each direction. As you become more confident, try turning your upper body in the direction you are pulling, without moving your hips.

Back Stretches

These stretches are excellent for people with lower back pain and are a good way to finish off an exercise session when you've been working on your back muscles. Make sure that you lift your legs to your chest one at a time and lower them separately at the end, or you could strain your lower back.

STRETCH I

❶ Lie on your back with your knees bent, feet on the floor in line with your hips, hands resting on your lower abdomen, and elbows on the floor. Support your head with a small pillow or a paperback book. Lift your right knee up toward your chest and hold it with your right hand. Then lift your left leg up and hold it with your left hand. Your knees should be roughly in line with your shoulders. Keep your elbows wide and shoulders relaxed into the floor. Breathe in.

❷ As you breathe out, engage your abdominals and pull your right knee toward you, keeping your chest soft and relaxed. Hold for a few seconds, then release.

❸ Pull your left knee toward you, then release.

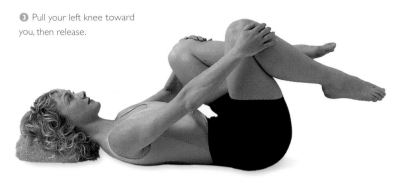

❹ Pull both knees together, keeping them slightly apart. Put one foot down carefully, then the other.

STRETCH 2

❶ Kneel on all fours with your hands slightly in front of your shoulders and your knees beneath your hips. Breathe in.

❷ As you breathe out, engage your abdominals and move your bottom back toward your heels, lowering your upper body until your forehead is on the floor. Slide your hands out in front of you as far as you can, feeling the stretch right through your spine. Breathe in and rest in this position for ten seconds.

Back Stretches

ALEXANDER REST

This resting position, developed by Frederick Alexander (1869–1955), is excellent for aligning the spine and relaxing the muscles. Lie on your back with your knees bent, feet parallel and hip-width apart. Rest the back of your head on a book so that your neck is straight. Experiment with different thicknesses of books until you find one that supports your head so that your neck is completely straight: it could be anything from a thin paperback to a chunky telephone directory. Place your hands on your lower abdomen, with your elbows resting on the floor. Breathe calmly, feeling gravity relax your muscles into the floor while your spine is held completely straight. Stay in the rest position for up to 20 minutes to get the full benefit.

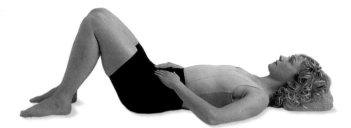

Questions & Answers

Q I know I should avoid twisting when I lift something. Are there any other day-to-day movements that could be harmful to my back?

A Never pick something up with straight legs; always bend your knees, no matter how small the object is. Avoid carrying children on one side all the time; alternate sides. Don't push heavy furniture; get someone to help. And watch out for supermarket trolleys with faulty wheels, which force you to twist and push at the same time.

Q I work in a desk job and get recurrent lower back pain. Should I support my lower back with a cushion while I'm working?

A Check your chair is the correct height so both feet rest on the ground. Make sure your computer and telephone are positioned so that you don't need to twist around to reach them, and that your desk is at the correct height. It is a good idea to support your lower back with a small cushion. *See also the advice on sitting, on page 23.*

Q It's more difficult to hold my abdominal muscles when lying on my front. Is there a special way of doing it?

A It is more difficult because the abdomen falls forward and you are working against gravity to pull it in, but you should just keep practicing until the area gets stronger. Practice your static abs in all the different positions listed on pages 51–53.

 Q I have sciatica in my right hip. Which exercises should I avoid and which ones are useful for alleviating it?

 A First of all, consult your physician to see what is causing it. Follow all the postural rules to help relieve strain on your lower back. Avoid movements that arch your back, like the Cobra, and be very careful when doing hamstring stretches. Static abs and very small pelvic tilts will help.

Q My arms don't seem to be strong enough to do the Cat and Dog exercises. They ache when I try to support my weight in this way. Should I skip them for now?

A If your wrists feel uncomfortable, rest your hands on a rolled-up towel. Don't lock your elbows. There are exercises to strengthen the arms on pages 151–57, so try these and persevere with the Cat and the Dog. If you feel insecure with the Dog, just stretch out an arm first, then a leg, before you do them both together.

Q When an exercise requires you to lie on your front, should you breathe into your back, as described in the breathing lesson?

 A No, you should breathe into your lungs, as in the scarf exercise (see page 32). Practice breathing while lying on your front with your hands placed on your ribs. They should move in and out.

The Upper Torso

Give your shoulders a little massage. Do the muscles feel smooth and lean, or bunched up and hard, as if there are rocks inside them? Sit up straight in a chair and turn your upper body to the left and then to the right. Can you go as far in both directions? Can you feel any stiffness in your shoulderblades? If you can't, you are in the minority. Tension in the upper back and shoulders is endemic in the modern world. This area tenses automatically when people are stressed or anxious, or if something takes them by surprise. Our shoulders hunch forward when we lean over a desk to read, or do the dishes, or drive a car, or sit in a badly designed seat at the theater.

The first chapter explained the correct way to sit, with your feet firmly on the ground, your back straight, and the backs of your thighs resting on the chair. If you consistently slouch or sit incorrectly, the muscles in the middle of the back ride upward, causing stiffness in the neck and shoulders. The chest collapses forward, inhibiting

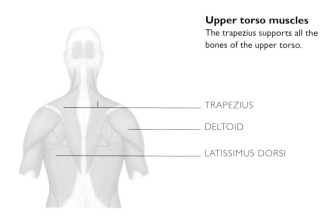

Upper torso muscles
The trapezius supports all the bones of the upper torso.

TRAPEZIUS

DELTOID

LATISSIMUS DORSI

Shoulderblades
A range of muscle groups assist the movement of the shoulderblades.

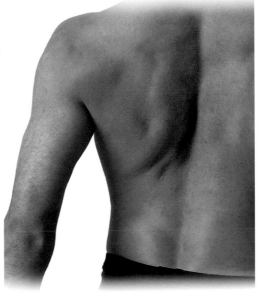

breathing, and there are knock-on effects for the balance and alignment of the rest of the body. Check your posture right now, as you're reading this page. Are you hunched over, or is your spine straight and your head held up?

The trapezius is a large diamond-shaped muscle stretching from the back of the head to midway down the spine and across the tops of the shoulderblades out to the collarbones. It helps to support the neck and head, it anchors the shoulderblades, and it is used when we raise our arms. If the lower part of the diamond shape is not held in position, it can ride up and cause the bunching effect many people experience in their shoulders. In this section, we will look at a variety of exercises for strengthening the trapezius and latissimus dorsi muscles, thus enabling the upper trapezius and other muscles of the neck and shoulders to be freer. We will also run through a series of exercises to strengthen the arm, shoulder, and chest muscles, so consult your physician first if you have problems with any of these areas.

Loosening Up

If your shoulder muscles are very taut just before an exercise session, a brief massage is a good idea—otherwise the muscles could tighten further when you start to work them. If you don't have someone to do this for you, you can rub your own shoulders for 30 seconds or so before each session.

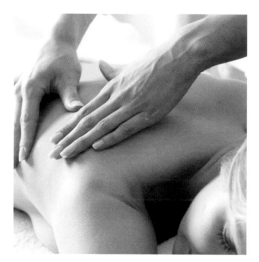

The benefits of massage
Gentle massage can release blockages in tight muscles.

ELBOW CIRCLES
Do this sitting or standing. Place your fingertips on top of your shoulder joints and slowly draw circles in the air with your elbows. Don't make the circles too big; the joints shouldn't click or feel strained, and your shoulders shouldn't hunch. Imagine you are gently oiling the insides of the shoulder joints. Do five circles with your elbows moving forward and another five moving backward.

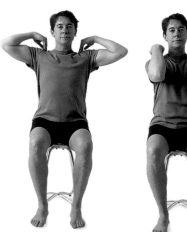

ARM CIRCLES

Stand with your feet comfortably apart, one foot in front of the other and your front leg bent. Lean forward to rest your right hand on the back of a chair. Let your left arm hang loosely down and circle it in both directions. Repeat with the right arm.

SLIDING THUMB

Standing or sitting straight, try and slide your left thumb up between your shoulderblades. Now repeat with the right thumb. Is it harder on one side than the other? Make a note of the side that is stiffer.

Working the Lats

Pages 108–9 explained how to do sitting lats. The following exercises also work the lats, but in different ways. Always ensure that your shoulders and neck aren't tensing up; shake your head lightly to make sure that the neck remains loose. Imagine a triangle running between your shoulders with its apex in the middle of your chest, and feel this triangle expanding as you open your palms outward.

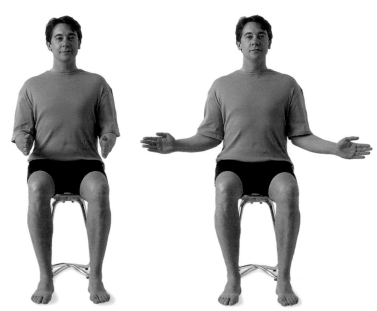

❶ Sit in a chair or on a stool with your back straight and your feet on the floor. Bend your elbows at an angle of 90° and position them slightly in front of your shoulders. Don't push them into your waist; there should be a gap where the waist curves inward. Turn your palms so they are facing each other. Breathe in.

❷ As you breathe out, engage your abdominals, slightly pull down your shoulderblades to engage the lats, and slowly open your palms outward, keeping your elbows in the same position. Your upper arms will rotate and your chest will widen, but the back muscles should be doing the work. Go as far as you can, then breathe in to return to the starting position. Repeat ten times.

VARIATION 1—PALMS UP

Do the same exercise with your palms facing upward. You should feel this working a slightly different part of the back muscles. Remember that your elbows are like pivots; they shouldn't move themselves.

VARIATION 2—PALMS DOWN

Do the same exercise with your palms facing downward. Like variation 1, this will work a different area of the back. Turn your head to make sure that your neck isn't tensing.

VARIATION 3—ELBOW BACK

With your palms facing down, do Variation 2, but before returning to the starting position, lift your elbows outward until your forearms are parallel, then slide them back. It can help to watch yourself in the mirror to make sure you aren't moving your shoulders, which would mean you were letting your upper trapezius muscle do the work. During the pulling back movement, you should be able to feel your lats engaging, just under your shoulderblades, as well as the rhomboids, the muscles between your shoulderblades.

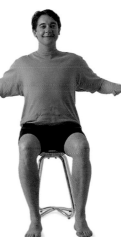

Cossack Arms

Once again, be careful that you don't feel any tension in your neck or shoulders. Imagine that your arms are weightless and visualize your back muscles doing the work. If you have problems with this exercise, try variation 1, in which your arms rest on a tabletop.

❷ Breathe out, engage your abdominals, pull down your shoulderblades gently to engage the lats, and slowly turn your upper body to the right. Your arms will travel around slightly farther than your chest, but make sure your shoulders are relaxed and your spine straight, with your hips facing forward. Imagine your upper body twisting around your spine from the waist upward. Don't worry if you can't turn very far in the beginning.

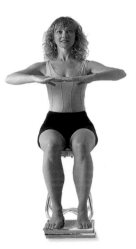

❶ Sit straight with your elbows bent and your feet and knees hip-width apart. Then with your palms facing downward, touch your fingertips together just in front of your breastbone, about 6 in. (15 cm) away. Breathe in.

❸ Breathe in to move back to the starting position and breathe out to turn to the left this time. Repeat five times in each direction. Keep your hips and knees still.

VARIATION 1—ARMS ON A TABLE

If you find this exercise difficult, try resting your arms on a table or surface that is about chest height. Twist around and as you reach the farthest you can go, extend the leading arm behind you.

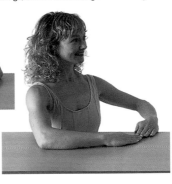

VARIATION 2—WITH EXERCISE BALL

Try performing the same movement while holding onto an exercise ball.

VARIATION 3—AN EXTRA BREATH

Once you have mastered the basic exercise, take an extra breath after step 2 and see if you can turn around just a little bit farther.

The Windmill

Do this very slowly and make sure you get the breathing pattern correct. You breathe in as you bring your arms up to the vertical and out as they move down again. The movement should be smooth and flowing, like the paddles of the windmill the exercise is named after.

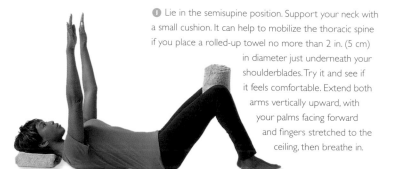

❶ Lie in the semisupine position. Support your neck with a small cushion. It can help to mobilize the thoracic spine if you place a rolled-up towel no more than 2 in. (5 cm) in diameter just underneath your shoulderblades. Try it and see if it feels comfortable. Extend both arms vertically upward, with your palms facing forward and fingers stretched to the ceiling, then breathe in.

❷ As you breathe out, engage your abdominals and then take your right arm back toward the floor beside your head and your left arm forward to the floor by your hip. Make sure your arms don't curve in or stray outward, and take them only as far as is comfortable. Don't let your back arch.

❸ Breathe in as you bring both arms up to center again, then breathe out as you move your left arm to the floor beside your head and your right arm down beside your hip. Repeat this ten times, keeping your chest soft.

MAKING A CIRCLE

① Adopt the same starting position as for the basic windmill, with your arms straight up and palms facing forward. Breathe out, bringing your right arm back to the floor beside your head and the other down to the floor by your hip, then continue the movement outward to make a circle on the floor. Feel the stretch.

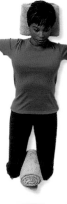

② When both arms reach shoulder height, pause and breathe in, turning your right hand palm downward and your left hand palm upward.

③ Breathe out to complete the circle, then breathe in as your raise your arms back to vertical again. Next time, start with your left arm going backward and your right forward. Repeat ten times in each direction.

TAKE CARE

Whatever you do, don't strain your shoulder joints. These are the most vulnerable joints in the body and they can take a long time to heal after injury. If your shoulder "clicks" or feels uncomfortable while doing this exercise, try making the circle a little smaller. If you still find it difficult, you could try the exercise standing up.

Upper Torso Release

This is a great way of loosening up tight shoulderblades. While the Windmill moves them up and down, this is a side-to-side movement that releases the muscles between them. Try to keep your forearms in a straight line throughout.

1 Lie on your back with your knees bent, feet on the floor. Support your head with a small cushion and relax your shoulders into the floor. Clasp your lower arms together and hold them just above your breastbone. Breathe in.

2 As you breathe out, engage your abdominals and lower your right elbow to the floor by your right side, letting the left arm follow. Keep your head straight and your shoulders relaxed. Feel the stretch through your left shoulder.

3 Breathe in to come up through the center and breathe out to stretch to the other side until your left elbow is resting on the floor by your left side. Repeat ten times in a smooth, continuous movement, keeping your forearms straight.

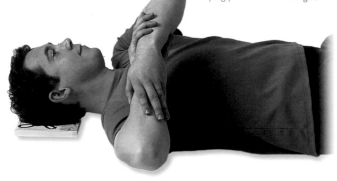

MAKING A CIRCLE

❶ Adopt the same starting position and lower your right elbow to the floor, then slowly continue around in a circle on the floor above your head, clasping your lower arms.

❷ Breathe in as you bring your arms back up to the starting position, then repeat the movement, making a circle in the opposite direction. Continue for ten continuous circles, alternating the direction each time.

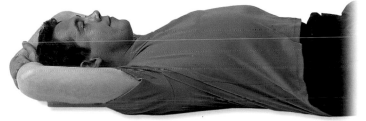

VARIATION—CHANGING THE GRASP

If it feels very tight when you clasp your forearms, try clasping your wrists instead. Alternatively hold a tape or CD in front of you to do the exercise.

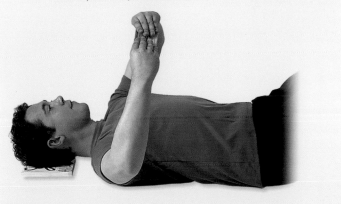

Shoulder Release

These exercises are great for opening up the shoulderblades and stretching the insides of the arms. In the supine version, you won't be able to reach the opposite palm unless one of your arms is substantially longer than the other, but that is what you are aiming for! The version lying on your side is more of a stretch, because your arm travels down to the floor behind you. You may not be able to reach all the way back at first, but after a few weeks, the mobility of your shoulders will increase.

SUPINE

❶ Lie on your back with your legs straight and parallel, hip-width apart. Your arms should rest straight out to the sides at shoulder height, with your palms facing upward.

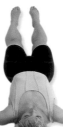

❷ Breathe in and bring your left arm up across your chest.

❸ Breathing out, engage your abdominal muscles and turn your upper body as you slide your left hand down your right arm toward your right palm. Turn your head in line with your arm, looking at your hands. Go as far as you can without moving your hips off the floor. Return to the starting position and repeat five times on each side.

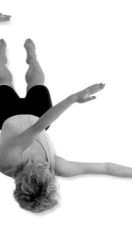

LYING ON YOUR SIDE

❶ Lie on your side in the fetal position, with your knees
and hips bent at 90°. Make sure your feet are together and
that your hip bones are directly on top of each
other. Stretch your arms out in front of
you, with your palms together.

❷ Breathe in and then, as you
breathe out, engage your abdominal
muscles and lift the top arm slowly
upward toward the ceiling and back
over your upper body.

❸ Let your head follow your
arm around as it descends
to the floor behind you. Your
shoulder should come back
to the floor, while your hips and
knees stay in position. Breathe
in and hold the stretch for five
seconds, then breathe out as
you return to the starting
position. Repeat five times
on each side.

MAKING A CIRCLE

❶ Adopt the same starting
position, lying on your side with
your palms together. Breathe in
and, as you breathe out, draw a
circle above your head with
your top arm. Stretch right
around until your fingers are
just beyond the opposite
shoulder. Stop and breathe in.

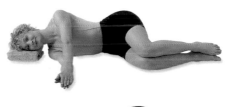

❷ Breathe out as you continue
the circle around the other
side, then bring your arm back
across your body to the
starting position. Repeat five
times in each direction.

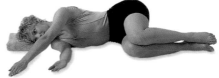

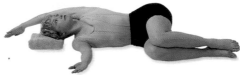

Crawling Up the Wall

You could do this in front of a mirror if you have one large enough. Otherwise, a wall is fine. Do the exercise very slowly, feeling the different back muscles working as you move your fingers around.

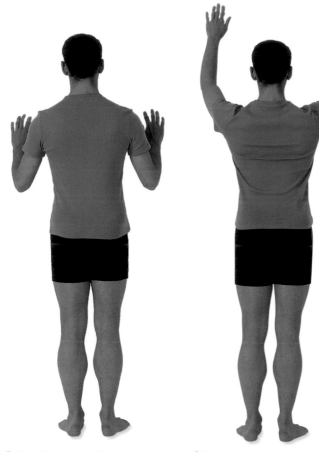

❶ Stand facing a wall with your feet directly under your hips and your back straight. When you bend your elbows, your fingers should be able to touch the wall. Breathing in, start crawling your fingers up the wall.

❷ Stop when your arms are straight. Make sure you don't lock your elbows or lift your shoulders.

3 As you breathe out, gently press your fingertips onto the wall and slide them around, as if drawing large semicircles on the wall on each side. Stretch as far as you can, while keeping your neck and shoulders relaxed.

TAKE CARE

If you have neck or shoulder problems, take a step backward to make the circle smaller. Stop at any time if it feels uncomfortable, but complete all the sections of the circle that you are capable of.

4 When your arms reach the level of your hips, turn the palms backward and gently press them behind your hips, engaging the lats. Repeat the circle five times.

Side Stretches

All of these stretches use an "anchor" of some kind to prevent you from stretching too far and hurting yourself. For the first version, use an upright dining room chair with no arms and a ladder back that is easy to hold onto. Before trying the stretch, make sure you are sitting properly in the chair, with your weight evenly distributed across the triangle shape in your feet, as described on page 14.

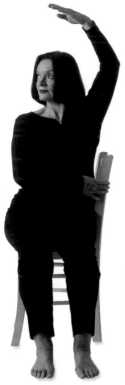

❶ Sit sideways on the chair, with the chair back to your left side. Make sure your hips are square and your feet are facing forward, hip-width apart. Hold onto the back with your right hand and curve your left arm above your head. Stop and check that your spine is straight and your shoulders relaxed. Breathe in.

❷ As you breathe out, engage your abdominal muscles, turn your head to the right, and stretch over to the right, so that your left elbow rises toward the ceiling. Look in the direction of the stretch. Your right hand holding the chair back will limit the distance you can stretch.

❸ Breathe in to return to the center. Repeat on the other side. Do five repetitions in each direction.

VARIATION I—HAND UNDER ARM

① Sit with the chair back behind you and place your left hand on your ribs, with the heel of the palm as close to the left armpit as possible. Breathe in.

② As you breathe out, engage your abdominals and turn your head to the left, then stretch over to the left. You won't be able to stretch as far as you did in the first version, as your hand will act as a brake. This variation stretches the thoracic spine, while the first version stretches the waist. Breathe in to return to the center. Repeat the stretch five times on each side.

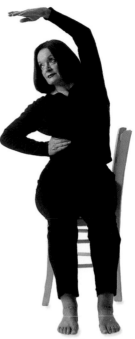

VARIATION 2—USING AN ANCHOR

① Stand straight with your feet slightly apart and one hand holding onto a doorknob, chair, or other well-anchored piece of furniture that is about 12 in. (30 cm) away from you sideways on. Breathe in.

② As you breathe out, stretch your other hand over your head toward the door, turning your head in the direction of the door. Keep your hips facing straight forward. Breathe in to return to the center and repeat five times on each side.

TAKE CARE

Make sure you turn your head to look in the direction you are moving, away from the stretch. Do these very gently if you have neck problems.

Shoulder Stretch

1 Stand straight in a door frame or at a corner where you can lean your arm against the wall on one side. Your palm should press the wall in line with your shoulder. Breathe in.

2 Engage your abdominals, then press into the wall and walk your feet around in the other direction, feeling the stretch in your shoulder. Breathe in to return to the center. Repeat five times on each side.

Lying Pecs

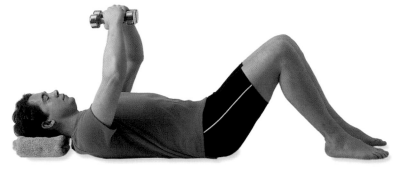

❶ Lie on your back with your knees bent and feet on the floor, with a small cushion supporting your head. Curve your arms up above your chest so that your fingertips are touching (or, if you are using weights, they are touching), holding your elbows wide to form a circle. Keep your shoulders relaxed. Breathe in.

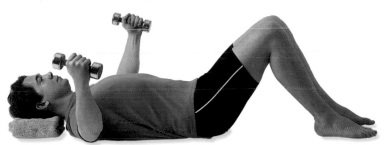

❷ As you breathe out, engage your abdominals and open your arms out to the sides, keeping the same curve. Start with a small movement and build up until you can touch your hands to the floor on either side.

❸ Breathe in as you bring your hands back together, closing the circle again. Repeat ten times.

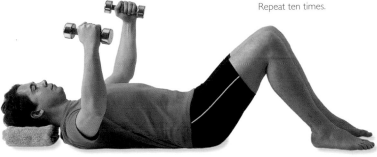

Pillow Squeeze

This is a good exercise to try if your serratus anterior muscles are weak. You should be able feel the shoulderblades being drawn forward, away from the spine, while your chest stays open and relaxed. You'll need a soft pillow.

❶ Sit straight in a chair with a pillow folded in half under one arm and held between your ribs and your elbow. Breathe in.

❷ As you breathe out, squeeze the pillow. Hold for a count of five, then relax. Repeat ten times on each side.

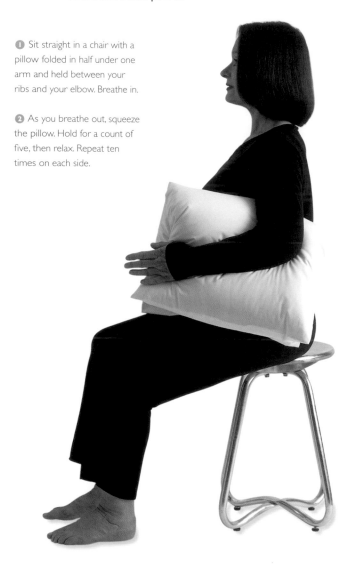

Questions & Answers

Q Why does my upper back feel stiff when I wake in the morning?

A Check the height of your pillow. If it is too high, it can cause a stiff neck and upper back. It should support the head so that the spine remains in a straight line all the way up. Also, check that your mattress isn't so soft that your back is "dipping" down into it.

Q I have a lot of paperwork in my job and always have aching shoulders at the end of the day from bending over my desk. But how else can I do my job?

A Make sure you sit correctly in your chair, with your feet on the floor and thighs at right angles to your lower leg. After 20 or 30 minutes, get up and walk around. You can buy tilted drawing boards for reading at a desk, which mean you don't have to bend your neck forward. When you are reading a book, lift it up to eye level.

Q I thought I was reasonably fit, but I seem to have a very limited range of movement when I try to do the circle versions of the Windmill or shoulder releases.

A  It could just be that your muscles are tight, in which case you should keep trying the exercises without forcing anything. If there is severe pain, though, you might have frozen shoulder—a condition caused by the inflammation of the joint lining—and you should seek medical advice.

Q My 14-year-old son complains of neck and shoulder stiffness. Should I introduce him to some basic Pilates exercises?

A At that age, it's possible he has just had a growth spurt, and he should exercise with caution. Work on correct postural alignment with him and try a few simple exercises like the basic Windmill and sitting lats to release the stiffness.

The Neck

The neck carries a lot of very important structures: the spinal cord, which transmits nerve impulses to and from the brain; the windpipe, which takes air to and from the lungs; the esophagus, which transports food and drink to the stomach; and the major blood vessels, which supply the head. As well as this, the neck has to support the weight of the head—11–13 pounds (5–6 kg) on average—and enable it to move up and down and from side to side. It's no wonder that neck problems can be so debilitating and capable of causing such a wide range of symptoms. Tension in the neck muscles can constrict the blood vessels, causing dizziness and fainting; it can cause headaches and migraines; if nerves become trapped, there can be tingling and numbness down the arms and into the fingers, along with nausea and shortness of breath.

The three main muscle groups worked on in this lesson are the sternocleidomastoids, running from the ear down to the base of the neck, which enable you to turn your head and pull it forward; the levator scapulae, which run from the top of the spine to the shoulderblade; and the top part of the trapezius muscle, also discussed

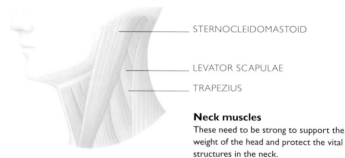

STERNOCLEIDOMASTOID

LEVATOR SCAPULAE

TRAPEZIUS

Neck muscles
These need to be strong to support the
weight of the head and protect the vital
structures in the neck.

Telephone strain
This makes the neck
muscles contract on
one side and stretch
on the other.

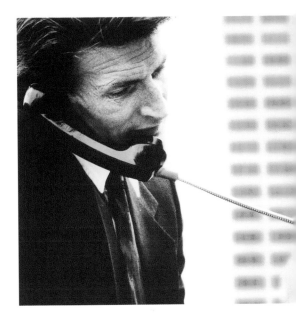

in the Upper Torso section. The exercises in this section will help you

to release tension in the neck muscles, and lengthen, strengthen, and

mobilize them while supporting the weight of the head.

If you have neck problems, always seek medical advice before trying

any kind of exercise. Ask your physician whether your neck requires

mobilization or stabilization and, if it's the latter, concentrate on the

isometric exercises on pages 144–45. Stop immediately if you

experience any pain, dizziness, or tingling in the arm or hand. Perform

the movements slowly and carefully to avoid placing any stress on

the spinal joints or damaging the neck muscles. Pilates exercises are

designed so that the weight of the head is always supported in some

way while the neck muscles are stretched, to avoid overstraining them.

Be careful to apply this principle to other activities in everyday life as

well; see the "Don't Ever" box on page 140.

Correcting Posture

You will avoid neck problems only by correcting your overall posture and building core stability, because any misalignments farther down the body will have a knock-on effect on the neck. If your knees, your pelvis, or your lower back are misaligned and the abdominals are weak, then your neck will be affected sooner or later. When held correctly, the weight of the head should be in line with the torso and supported on the spine. The chin must be held level and slightly back, rather than jutting forward. It can be useful to imagine a piece of string running through the spinal column and emerging through the crown of the head; pull the imaginary string straight and your spine will be in the correct alignment. When you bend your head forward, the muscles at the front of the neck shorten and those in the back of the neck tighten.

If you consistently hold your head forward or to one side during the day, or if your pillows don't support your head correctly in bed, the muscles will shorten on the side you bend toward and tighten on the other side.

DON'T EVER

● Try to release tension by circling your head around unsupported

● Make any rapid, jerky movements with your head

● Hold a telephone between your ear and your shoulder

● Carry heavy loads in a shoulder bag

● Try to force your neck farther than it will go comfortably

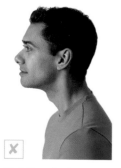 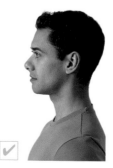

Holding the head
The chin should not jut forward.

Figure Eight

This is a very tiny movement that stretches the muscles supporting the very top of your neck, just where it reaches your skull. It can help to relieve tension headaches.

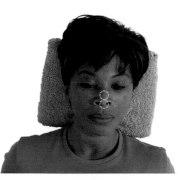

❶ Lie on your back with your knees bent, feet slightly apart, and arms by your sides, and support your head on a paperback book or folded towel. Look straight up at the ceiling. Try to imagine that there is a blackboard just above your nose, and that you have chalk on the end of your nose. What you have to do is draw a figure eight on the blackboard.

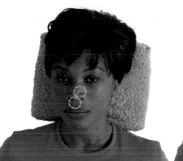

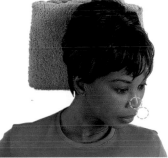

❷ Start in the middle and draw the first loop. As you go outward, your nose will have to lift slightly so that it is still in touch with the blackboard. It is only a very small figure eight you are drawing—no longer than your nose!

❸ Come back to the middle, then draw your figure eight in the other direction. Do it very slowly and repeat four times in each direction, breathing naturally throughout.

TAKE CARE

The exercises on pages 141, 142, and 143 mobilize your neck and shouldn't be attempted if your physician has told you to stabilize it.

Chin to Chest

Usually you shouldn't sink your chin into your chest in Pilates movements. This exercise to stretch out your neck is the one exception to the rule. Keep your shoulders relaxed into the floor and don't contort your face or grit your teeth trying to pull farther than you can naturally go.

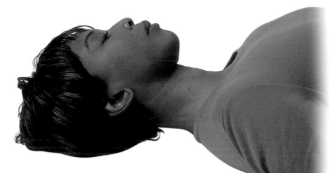

❶ Lie in the same position as for the Figure Eight, but without the book or towel under your head.

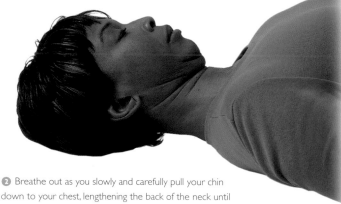

❷ Breathe out as you slowly and carefully pull your chin down to your chest, lengthening the back of the neck until you are almost flattening it against the floor. Imagine a stretch through the crown of your head. Hold for five seconds, then relax. Repeat five times.

Side to Side

If your neck starts to feel tight in the middle of the working day, this is a simple way to release the muscles—so long as you have a pillow or a folded towel on hand.

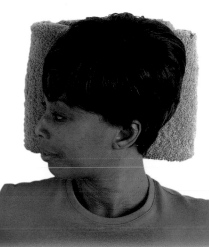

❶ Lie on your back with your knees bent and your arms by your sides. Support your head with a comfortable pillow or folded towel that holds your neck straight. Slowly let your head roll to the right, as far as it will go without straining. The weight of your head should control the movement.

❷ Return to the center, then roll to the left. Repeat five times.

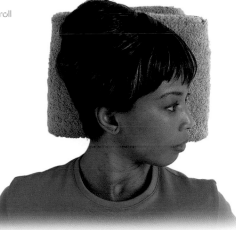

Isometric
Neck Exercises

Isometric is a technical term for a movement that contracts a muscle without shortening it. If you have neck problems, you should beware of any movements that shorten the muscles on one side without providing support for the weight of the head. The exercise on these pages is safe for anyone with neck pain. It can help to sit facing a mirror as you do the movements so you can check that you are keeping your head straight. Repeat each of the steps two or three times.

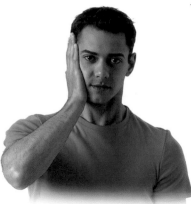

❶ Sit on a chair with your back straight and your feet on the floor. Check that your head is straight and your shoulders are level (if they're not, shrug them up to your ears and let them fall back naturally into position). Place your right hand against the right side of your face, with your palm on the cheek and fingers extending up to the forehead. Gently press against the side of your face, keeping your head straight. Hold for five seconds, then relax.

❷ Place your left hand on the left side of your face and press gently, feeling the neck muscles contract. Your head shouldn't move at all. Hold for five seconds and relax.

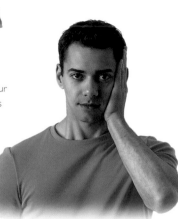

3 Make a loose fist and gently press it against your forehead, keeping your head straight. You'll feel the muscles on both sides of your neck. Hold for five seconds and relax.

4 Make a fist and press it upward under your chin. Don't engage your teeth or let your chin lift. You'll feel the muscles at the back of your neck. Hold for five seconds and relax.

Neck Stretches

You'll really feel these exercises stretching the muscles down the sides of the neck, over the shoulders, and right down through the arms. Be gentle; just go as far as you can without feeling any strain. Rather than actively "pulling" with your hand on top of your head, think of your arm being heavy and its weight pulling your head over.

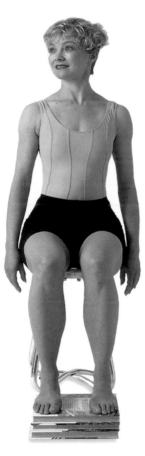

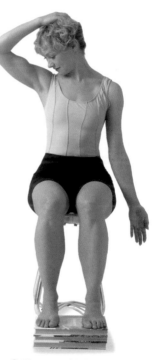

❶ Sit on a chair with your back straight and both feet on the floor. Turn your head slightly to the right.

❷ Place your right hand over the top of your head and gently pull it forward and farther to the right until you feel a stretch in the left side of your neck. Keep your nose in line with your elbow. Your shoulders should still be facing forward. Stretch your left arm down toward the floor with the palm facing backward, then rotate the palm outward until it faces forward. Hold the stretch for five seconds.

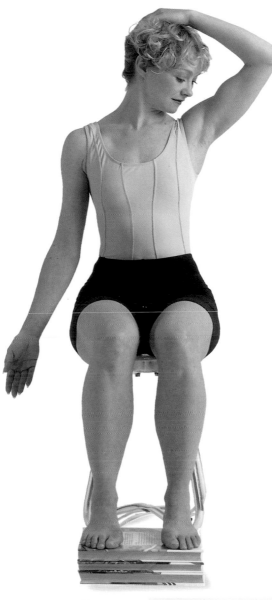

3 Repeat on the other side with your head turned slightly to the left, your left hand on top of your head, and your right arm stretching toward the floor. Hold for five seconds.

TAKE CARE

Don't attempt these neck stretches if your physician has told you to stabilize your neck rather than mobilize it.

Questions & Answers

Q When I hold my chin slightly back, as recommended for good posture, it feels uncomfortable in the sternocleidomastoid muscles.

A The chin should be held so that your ears are in line with your shoulder joints and hip joints. If you have been jutting your chin forward for a long time, it will feel odd to hold it back. You need to work on your back muscles to get the shoulders in the correct position first and then correct your head position.

Q I seem to strain my neck whenever I do abdominal curls. Should I work on strengthening the neck muscles to combat this?

A You need to support your head more during ab curls. Do only the version with the towel on page 61 and practice getting the energy down into your abdominals. You should also keep doing all the neck exercises in this lesson at every session.

Q I often wake up in the morning with a stiff neck. Can I do some neck exercises lying in bed?

A Your pillow may not be supporting your head properly, so check that first. Doing exercises in bed is not ideal, as the mattress may not be firm enough. If you feel stiff when you wake up, don't leap out of bed immediately; do some gentle stretches first. You could try the chin to chest and side to side neck exercises very carefully.

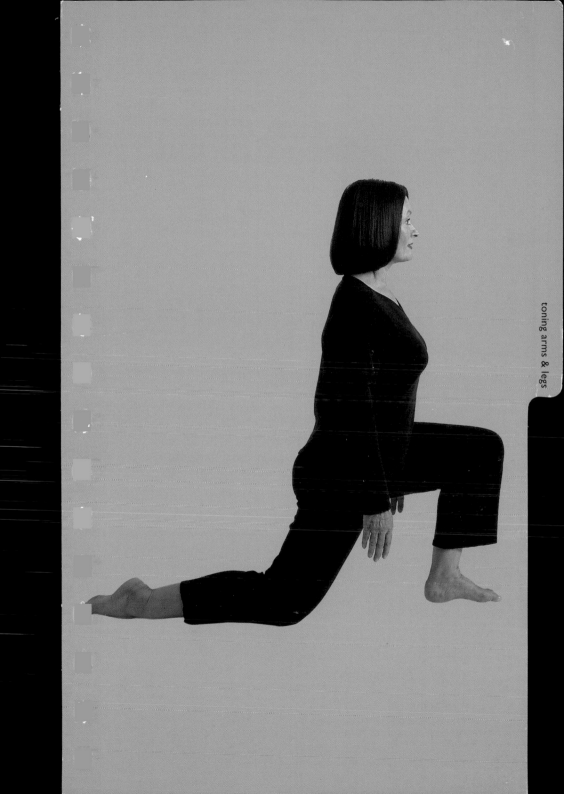

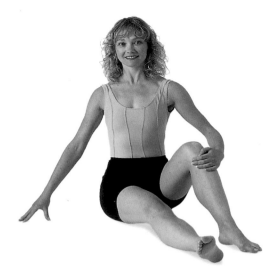

Toning Arms and Legs

It's important to keep the muscles of the arms and legs strong in order to protect their joints. We looked at the shoulder joint in the last chapter. Elbows and wrists can also become painful if they are repeatedly used with incorrect alignment, and knees are very complex joints, with a lot of structures that can be damaged. The thigh bone, kneecap, and lower leg bone are held together by various ligaments running down the sides and diagonally across the joint cavity. Field sports that involve running and turning quickly can cause damage to the ligaments and football and soccer players are particularly at risk from knee injuries because of the kicking movements. The exercises in this section focus on the muscles that stabilize the arm and leg joints, thus helping to prevent injuries.

Arms & Hands

Think of all the ways we use our arms: carrying heavy bags and suitcases, typing on a computer keyboard, answering the telephone, hugging friends and family, playing racket sports, and holding this book at an angle that allows you to read it! Arms have to perform a wider variety of functions than legs, and their joints require a greater range of movement. You can rotate your hand and forearm through almost 180 degrees at the elbow joint; try this by holding your bent elbows into your sides, with your palms facing upward in front of you, then turning the palms so they face down. The angle between your hand and forearm has a range of roughly 180 degrees as well. These movements are made possible by groups of tendons and ligaments stabilizing the joints, and many of the injuries to arm joints, such as tennis elbow or repetitive strain injury, occur when the tendons are strained.

You can help to protect yourself against strains by strengthening the muscles that keep the joints and tendons in correct alignment. The arm exercises on the following pages are all very simple, but double check you are lined up correctly before you start. Feel free to use hand weights to intensify the effects, but don't buy any that are heavier than roughly 1 pound (500g)—about the weight of a can of beans.

When you take your weight on your arms in exercises that require you to kneel on all fours, make sure your weight is evenly spread through the back and front of the arms. If you find this position puts strain on your wrists, try resting them on a rolled-up towel—or avoid these exercises until your muscles are stronger.

Working the Wrists

If you hold a lot of tension in your wrists, there are some simple movements you can use to release it.

Try resting your forearm on the arm of a chair, with your hand extending over the edge. Make a soft fist, then move your hand slowly up and down then from side to side. You can do this during the working day, perhaps after you have been typing or writing for a while.

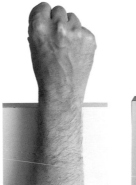
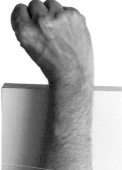

To strengthen the muscles in the wrists and the backs of the hands, clasp your hands together, using about 50 percent force, then slowly pull them apart, still clasping to resist the movement.

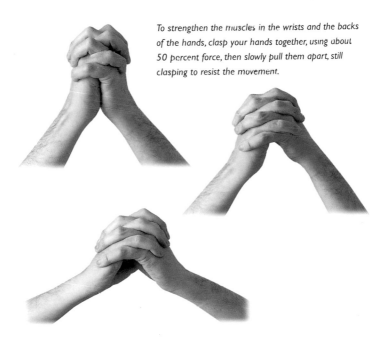

Arm Exercises

These are all quite simple movements, which strengthen the muscles through repetitions. When you are confident you can do them correctly, use light arm weights or hold a can of beans or some other object of similar weight while performing them. Increase the number of repetitions as you get stronger.

SITTING DELTOIDS

1 Sit straight in a stool or chair without arms, keeping your feet firmly on the floor, arms straight by your sides.

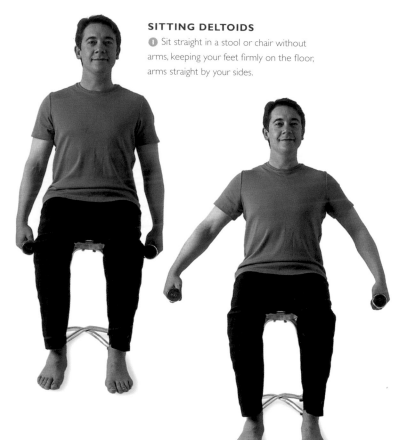

2 Breathe out, engage the abdominals, and lift your arms out to the side until they are slightly lower than shoulder level. Breathe in to return to the starting point.

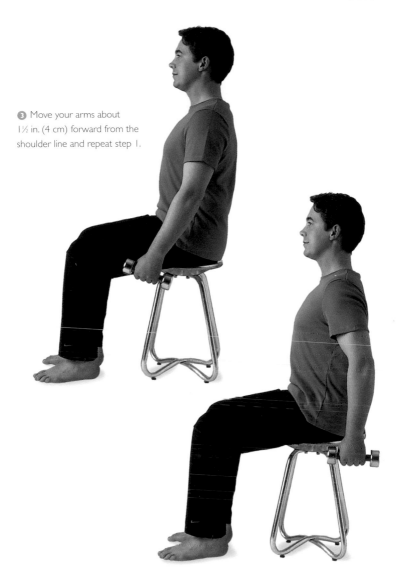

❸ Move your arms about 1½ in. (4 cm) forward from the shoulder line and repeat step 1.

❹ Move your arms about 1½ in. (4 cm) backward from the shoulder line and repeat step 1. Do five repetitions of all three movements to exercise different areas of the deltoids.

TAKE CARE

If you have elbow problems, such as tennis elbow, don't use weights for the arm exercises and limit the range of movement to avoid any strain.

Lying Triceps

It's important to keep your shoulders relaxed down into the floor so that you are not using shoulder or neck muscles for these movements. You should feel your triceps muscles working with the forearm that supports your elbow.

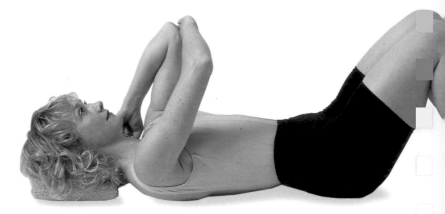

❶ Lie on your back with your knees bent, feet parallel and in line with your hips, and support your head with a small cushion. Bend your left elbow, so that the upper arm is perpendicular to the floor and your left hand is resting on your left shoulder. Place your right forearm behind your left elbow to support it, but keep your shoulders soft. Breathe in.

VARIATION 1—
SITTING AT A TABLE

If you find it difficult to hold your arm up in this position, you can do the exercise sitting up at a table with a box positioned under your upper arm so that it is parallel to the floor. Bend your elbow at an angle of 90° and then straighten your arm to work your triceps.

VARIATION 2—
OPENING THE ARM

Try bringing your hand toward the opposite ear—for example, your left hand toward your right ear—to use the triceps (and biceps) in a slightly different way.

❷ As you breathe out, engage your abdominals and straighten your elbow so that your upper arm is straight up, perpendicular to the floor. Breathe in to return to the starting point and do ten repetitions on each side.

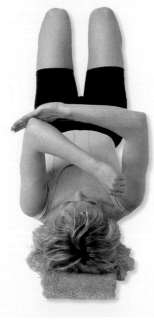

Sitting Biceps

Biceps and triceps are opposing muscle groups, so if you have been working one group, always follow up with the other to counterbalance. If your biceps are much stronger, do more repetitions of the triceps exercises.

1 Sit straight in a chair or stool with your feet on the floor, or resting on a pile of books if necessary to give an angle of 90° at hips and knees. Your arms should be straight by your sides so that the elbows are directly below your shoulders; don't let them tuck in at the waist. With your palms facing forward, make a soft fist (if you are holding weights, the weight should be at the front). Breathe in.

② As you breathe out, engage your abdominals and bend your elbow to raise your fist (or weight) toward your shoulder. Keep your elbow in the same position. Don't try to bend too far. Just go for a smooth, flowing movement.

③ Breathe in to straighten your arm again. Repeat ten times on each side, keeping your shoulders relaxed throughout.

Legs & Feet

Have a look at an old pair of your shoes. Where did they start to wear out first? If the heels are run down while the soles are more or less intact, you could be leaning your weight backward when standing and walking. If the soles are worn under the balls of your feet while the heels are fine, you may be leaning your weight forward. Are they worn on the inner sides or the outer sides? Is one shoe more worn than the other? As explained on page 14, your weight should be balanced through a triangle shape in your feet. If you are doing this, you would expect shoes to wear out equally across the soles and heels. However, if you wear shoes that are too loose, or cut too low over the arch, you could be tensing your feet muscles to keep them on as you walk, and if your shoes squash any part of your feet, they could be forcing your weight into different areas.

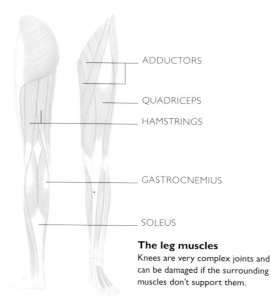

ADDUCTORS

QUADRICEPS

HAMSTRINGS

GASTROCNEMIUS

SOLEUS

The leg muscles
Knees are very complex joints and can be damaged if the surrounding muscles don't support them.

Stand up with bare feet and assess yourself again. Remember that your feet should be parallel and your kneecaps facing straight forward. Keep your knees slightly "soft," rather than locked. The extremes of bad posture include toes turned under like claws in people who are trying to balance their weight forward; toes bent upward in people who balance on their heels; bow legs in people who tend to roll onto the outsides of their feet; and knock-kneed postures in those who lean their feet to the insides. Do you have bunions, flat feet, or any other foot complaints? Any disorders will affect the way you balance your weight, thus knocking out the alignment of the knees and hips. On page 172 you will find an exercise to strengthen the feet muscles.

This section will exercise the quadriceps muscles, which run up the front of the thighs and enable you to straighten your knees; the hamstrings down the back of your thighs, which bend the knees; the adductor muscles in your inner thighs, which move your legs inward, and the outer thigh abductors, which move them outward. You should include some glute squeezes and hamstring curls in every Pilates session, because hamstrings are often weaker than other leg muscles, particularly the quadriceps.

Feet muscles
The feet muscles must be strong to support your weight evenly.

Balance Tests

It's one thing to keep your weight correctly aligned when standing, but when we are walking we need to balance our weight temporarily on one side then the other. The mechanics of walking are too complex to cover in this book, but it can be interesting to try a couple of simple tests to see how well your joints and muscles adapt to balancing your weight on each side.

Standing up, lift and bend your left leg and balance your weight on your right leg for a few seconds. How steady are you? Now try balancing your weight on your left leg. Is it easier on one side than the other? If so, it could mean that you need to work on strengthening the muscles more on the unsteady side.

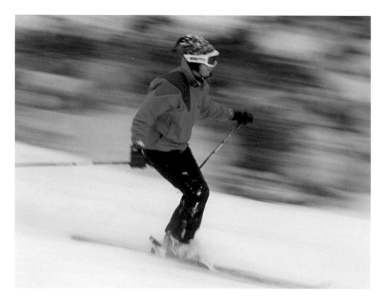

Skiing
Skiing can be very harmful to the knees because of the side-to-side movements;
skiers need very strong leg muscles to hold their knee joints in alignment.

Now try to walk in a straight line, placing each foot directly in front of each other, without looking down. Place your weight directly into the triangle shape in your feet rather than rolling from side to side. It's possible to do this without wobbling only if your pelvis and knee joints are correctly aligned, your leg muscles are in good condition, and you have strengthened the muscles responsible for good posture. In the Pilates studio, there is a low beam to practice walking along; it's harder than it looks!

TRY TO AVOID

● Crossing your legs

● Wearing shoes that don't hold your feet comfortably

● Sudden twists of the knee

● Sitting or kneeling with your knees turned in and feet splayed out to the sides

Balancing
When you stand on one foot, try to keep your hips level—don't lean into one side.

Shoes
It's important for the posture of the whole body to wear correctly fitting shoes that support your feet.

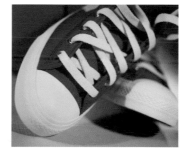

Inner Thighs—Sitting

If your inner thigh adductors aren't very strong, the quadriceps muscles may try to take over in these exercises. Wear close-fitting leggings or keep your legs bare so that you can actually see whether you are engaging the inner thigh muscles. They should be visible just above the inside of your knee. Rest your back against a chair (or an exercise ball, if you have one) to help keep it straight as you perform the movements. You can lean backward into it, but make sure you are engaging your stomach muscles.

❶ Sit on the floor with your back lightly resting against a chair and with your legs apart.

TAKE CARE

Don't take your leg inward past the center if you have had a hip replacement. If the backs of your thighs feel tight, do hamstring stretches to loosen them up (see page 177).

❷ Bend your left knee and stretch your right leg out to the side with the foot turned outward so your heel faces inward. The angle between your legs should just be as wide as you can manage comfortably—don't force it. Place your left hand on your left knee and let your right hand rest lightly on the floor by your side. Breathe in.

❸ As you breathe out, engage your abdominals, then slide your right foot inward without lifting it off the ground. Imagine you are spreading sand across the floor with your heel. Make sure the inner thigh muscles are doing the work. Take your leg inward until it is just past the center, then breathe in to return to the starting position. Repeat ten times.

❹ Change position so that your right knee is bent and your left leg stretched out on the floor. Do ten repetitions sliding your left leg across the floor.

VARIATION 1—WITH A WEIGHT

Place a weight on the ground just inside your heel and move it across the floor. You could use a can of soup or any other similar weight. However, you'll have to lean forward to return it to position after each movement. If you have a pair of strap-on ankle weights, they could be used instead.

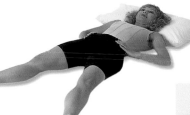

VARIATION 2—LYING DOWN

Do the exercise lying on your back with your neck and shoulders supported on cushions, your arms by your sides, and both legs stretched out to the sides. Alternate the legs, so you slide your right leg in and out then your left leg in and out. If you are using a weight, you could slide it from one leg to the other.

NOTE

This is one of the Pilates exercises where people can be surprised to discover asymmetries they weren't aware of before. Perhaps it's harder to turn your foot outward on one side, or maybe you manage the exercise easily with one leg but not the other. If this is the case, do more repetitions on the weaker side.

Outer Thighs— Lying on Side

Correct positioning is crucial for this exercise, or you could find that you're using the wrong muscles. Place the top hand on your outer thigh to feel the abductor muscles working. Always lengthen through your heel before lifting, and don't let your hips and shoulders roll forward or your waist fold inward.

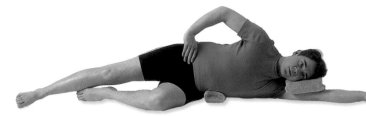

❶ Lie on your side with your back against a wall; this is not for support, but to make sure you lie in a straight line. Place a small cushion or rolled-up towel under your waist. Bend the bottom leg to make angles of 90° at your hip and knee. Stretch the bottom arm under your head, placing a cushion or folded towel between your upper arm and head. Place the fingers of the top hand lightly on the floor in front of you, or rest them on your outer thigh to check that you are using the correct muscles. Breathe in.

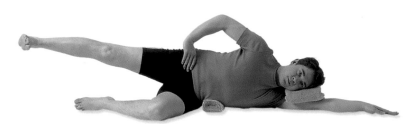

❷ Breathe out, engage your abdominals, then stretch your top leg down through the heel and lift it upward. Make sure your waist doesn't drop down; the leg should do all the work. Lift only as far as you can go without sinking your waist; it's more about lengthening than lifting. Return to the starting position and repeat five times. Then turn onto your other side and repeat five times.

Take plenty of time to check
your alignment before you begin
this exercise. Run through the
following checklist:
● Are your shoulder joints
directly on top of each other?
● Are your hip bones lined
up on top of each other?
● Are you lying in a straight line?
● Are your waist and neck
supported in such a way that the
spine is held straight?

CAUTION

If you have lower back pain, it is
imperative that your abdominals are
strong enough to support your torso
while you perform this exercise. You can
curve the body slightly to support the
lower back; experiment to see what
works for you. If you feel any twinges,
stop immediately and don't try it again
until you have done more work on
your core stability.

DOUBLE LEG LIFTS

This is an advanced movement. You shouldn't try it until you are confident that your core stability is strong and you can manage the outer thigh lifts easily. Don't worry if you wobble during the lift: making adjustments to correct your balance works a range of muscles at the same time.

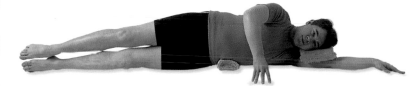

① Lie on your side with your back against a wall and both legs straight. Place a cushion between your lower arm and your head to support your neck and another cushion or rolled-up towel under your waist. Your feet, knees, and hips should all be parallel and facing forward—run through the checklist above left. Rest the fingers of your top arm lightly on the floor in front for balance. Breathe in.

② As you breathe out, engage your abdominals and stretch both legs before you lift them. Keep the lift quite low and don't try to hold it for long. Return your legs to the floor. Repeat five times on each side.

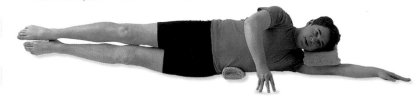

Inner Thighs—
Lying on Side

For this exercise, you adopt a similar starting position to the outer thigh lifts. Make sure you straighten downward through your heel before lifting the lower leg to engage the inner thigh muscles.

● Lie on your side with your back against a wall, using small cushions under your waist and between your head and lower arm. Curl your top leg over a pile of cushions, arranged to support it so there are angles of 90° at the knee and hip, but the knee is raised above the ground. Keep your lower leg straight. Make sure your shoulders are lined up and that your hip bones are directly on top of each other. Place the fingers of your top hand lightly on the floor in front, but be careful not to lean into them. Breathe in.

CHECKLIST

Once again, correct alignment is crucial,
so run through the checklist:
● Are your shoulder joints
directly on top of each other?
● Are your hip bones lined
up on top of each other?
● Are you lying in a straight line?
● Are your waist and neck
supported in such a way that the
spine is held straight?

CAUTION

If your inner thighs are unused to
exercise, work slowly and build the
strength gradually. It's only a small lift.
You'll feel the muscles working when
you're just an inch or so off the floor.

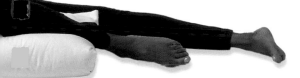

❷ As you breathe out, engage your abdominals, then
lengthen the lower leg down through the heel and lift it
off the floor, feeling your inner thigh working. Hold for
4 seconds, making sure your shoulders and hips don't roll
forward. Lower your leg. Repeat five times on each side.

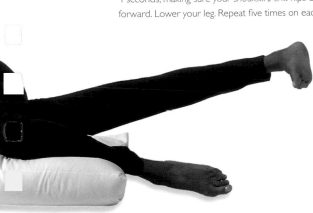

The Shell

Imagine a giant clam opening and closing its shell. In this exercise, your legs are like the two sides of the shell and the squeezing of the gluteus maximus muscles slowly opens them up. This squeeze works farther to the outsides of the glutes than the glute squeezes on pages 80–83, and you'll also feel it down the backs of your thighs.

① Lie on your side with your back against a wall and curl up your knees. Use a small cushion to support your waist, and place another cushion between your head and your lower arm. Rest the fingers of the top arm lightly on the floor in front of you, but don't lean into it. Check that your feet, hips, and shoulders are lined up. Breathe in.

VARIATION—WITH A PILLOW

To make this exercise work with more intensity, place a pillow between your feet.

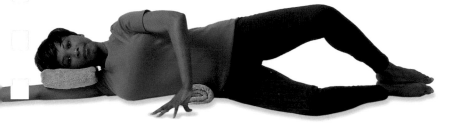

2 As you breathe out, engage your abdominals and then gently squeeze your glutes, using the movement to open your thighs as far as you can. Keep your hips and feet in the same positions. You'll feel it in the back of your thighs just under your bottom. Breathe in to return to the starting position. Repeat five times on each side.

Quadriceps

Whenever you do quadriceps exercises, counterbalance them by doing some hamstring curls (*see pages 84–85*) as well. In most people, the quads are fairly strong already since they are used for so many day-to-day activities. Make sure your kneecaps are facing straight forward before you start. You'll have to experiment with cushions or pillows to make the triangular supports needed.

❶ Arrange a cushion or rolled-up towel to support your neck as you lie on your back. Then arrange a triangular pile of cushions so that your left knee lies on top and the back of your left thigh rests against them while your heel is on the floor. Your right leg should be alongside the cushion with the knee bent and the sole of the foot firmly placed on the floor. Keep your arms by your sides. Check your left knee is straight and in line with your hips, then breathe in.

❷ As you breathe out, engage your abdominals and lift your left foot, keeping it softly flexed. Straighten your knee until you feel the muscles at the front of your thigh (your quads) tighten, then lower your foot again, breathing in.

❸ Repeat five times with the left leg, then five times with the right. Gradually build up to more repetitions.

SITTING ON A TABLE

Choose a table or other flat surface that is high enough off the ground so that your feet don't touch the floor when you sit on it. Both quadriceps exercises can be done with light strap-on ankle weights, but try it without weights first of all until you are confident of the movements.

❶ Sit straight on the table with your hands resting lightly on either side of you. Place a rolled-up towel under your left thigh just above the knee. Make sure your kneecaps are facing straight forward. Breathe in.

❷ As you breathe out, engage your abdominals and raise your left foot upward, keeping the foot soft.

❸ When your knee is straight, point your foot and flex it.

❹ Breathe in as you lower your foot again. Repeat five times with the left leg, then five times with the right.

TAKE CARE

If you have knee problems, be very careful when doing quadriceps exercises. Make only very small movements and stop if it is uncomfortable.

Feet and Calves

Weaknesses in the feet and calf muscles will have a snowball effect throughout the body, knocking the knees and hips out of alignment, so do these strengthening exercises regularly.

DOMING THE FEET

This is a very simple exercise you can do during a spare moment. Repeat it frequently, especially if you have any problems with your feet. It is performed with bare feet.

❶ Sit with your back straight in a chair that is the right height so that your knees and hips are bent at angles of 90° and your feet rest firmly on the floor, hip-width apart. Make sure that your weight is evenly distributed across the triangle shape in your feet (see page 14).

❷ Slide your toes back while keeping your heels in the same position, so that the arches on top of your feet rise up into a "dome." Don't let your toes curl under. Hold for five seconds before returning to the starting position.

CALF RAISES

This is another exercise that you can do whenever you have time, to strengthen the calf muscles. It also helps the feet muscles, as you roll your weight up onto the balls of the feet, then slowly back down again.

❶ Stand straight, holding onto a door frame or resting the palms of your hands against a wall. Check your posture: head straight, shoulders back, feet parallel and slightly apart, and knees soft, not locked. Breathe in.

❷ As you breathe out, engage your abdominals, squeeze your buttocks, and slowly lift up onto the balls of your feet, feeling your calf muscles working. Hold for five seconds before breathing in and bringing your heels back down to the floor. Repeat ten times in a slow, flowing movement.

Plié

This is a Pilates exercise that is usually done on the studio equipment, but here I have converted it to use a wall. It works a whole range of muscle groups. Don't try it until your core stability is strong and you can confidently do all the other leg exercises in this lesson.

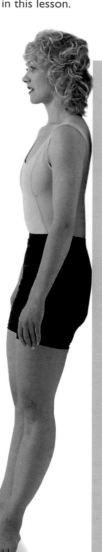

❶ Stand with your back against a wall or door frame. The distance between your heels and the wall or door frame should be roughly the same as the length of your feet. Rotate your feet outward slightly, keeping your heels close together but not quite touching, in a position that feels comfortable for you. Keep your shoulders relaxed.

TAKE CARE

Don't try this exercise if you have knee or hip problems. Stop immediately if it feels uncomfortable.

2 As you breathe in, engage your abdominals and slowly slide your back down the wall, letting your knees bend outward directly over your feet. Keep your heels on the floor. Don't lean forward or let your shoulders hunch or tense, and don't try to go too far down.

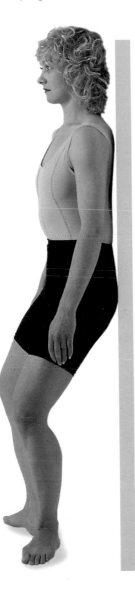

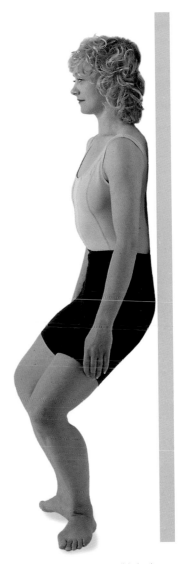

3 Stop, and breathe out as you slide back up the wall again. Repeat the plié five times. If you find this easy, try it with your legs farther apart, so there is a space about two-and-a-half times the length of your foot between your heels. You'll find this harder.

Leg Stretches

When you finish a session in which you have focused on leg exercises, it is a good idea to stretch out the muscles. You can use these stretches during a session as well, if any area feels tight.

QUADS

❶ Kneel on your left knee and bend your right leg forward with your foot on the floor, so that you have angles of 90° at each knee and at one hip. Keep your back straight and let your arms hang by your sides. Breathe in.

❷ Breathe out, engage your abdominals, and lean forward so the right knee bends outward directly over the top of the right foot. Keep your back and left thigh in a straight line. Repeat this stretch on the other side.

HAMSTRINGS

❶ Lie in the semisupine position. If you like, you can rest your head on a small cushion. Bend one leg up toward your chest, holding it just above the knee. Breathe in.

❷ As you breathe out, engage your abdominals and straighten the bent leg up to a vertical position, holding it with your hands. You could even pull it toward your head slightly—just stretch as far as you can manage, then lower it and repeat on the other side.

VARIATION—WITH A TOWEL

You can also do the hamstring stretch using a towel to pull your leg toward you. Loop it around the base of your foot and hold the ends. This also works in a sitting position, with one knee bent and one straight and a towel around the foot.

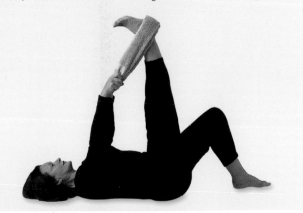

Leg Stretches

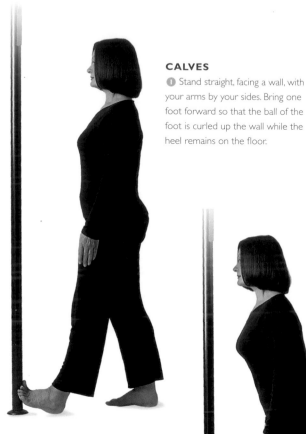

CALVES

① Stand straight, facing a wall, with your arms by your sides. Bring one foot forward so that the ball of the foot is curled up the wall while the heel remains on the floor.

② Keeping your back straight, lean forward as if to touch your forehead against the wall and feel the stretch in your calf. Repeat on the other side.

BACK OF KNEE

① Sit straight in a chair with one foot on the floor and the other leg straight in front of you with the heel resting on top of a pile of books or a box, about 6 in. (15 cm) off the floor. Rest your hands in the small of your back. Breathe in.

② As you breathe out, engage your abdominals and lean forward from the hips, keeping your back straight. You'll feel the stretch in the back of your knee. Sit up again and repeat on the other side.

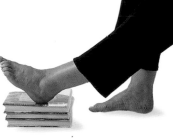

Questions & Answers

Q My mother taught me to rotate my feet around the ankles, forward and backward, so that I would have thin ankles. Is this a good idea?

A This is a good way of keeping the ankle joint mobile, rather than making the ankles thinner! Rotating the ankles strengthens a range of muscles that control the movements of the foot. This is another exercise you could do sitting at your desk during the day.

Q One of my knees makes a crunching sound when I bend it, as though there's a handful of gravel inside the joint. Will this do any harm?

A The crunching sound is caused by bits of calcified material that have come loose from the bone through wear and tear. So long as the crunching isn't painful, it won't do any harm. Always make sure you keep the knees in their correct alignment when bending, so there's no uneven pull on the muscles.

Q I cycle to work every day to keep fit. Does this use all the muscles in the legs or should I concentrate on some more than others when I do Pilates?

A Cycling uses the quads and the calves, so in your Pilates sessions you should do quad and calf stretches and work more on strengthening the hamstrings and inner thigh muscles.

Q Can you suggest any exercises I could do to keep the circulation going in my legs and feet during long-distance flights?

A Get up and move around. Don't spend too long just sitting in your seat. Do some calf stretches, dome your feet, and circle your ankles. Apart from the risks of deep vein thrombosis on long-distance flights, gentle stretches will help to prevent swollen ankles and feet.

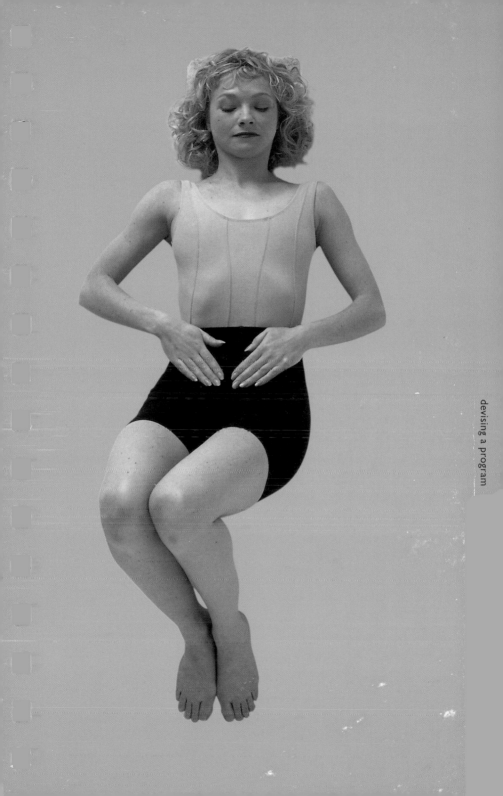

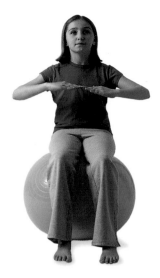

Devising a Program

This section shows you how to combine the exercises into routines, graduating through three stages: Gentle Beginnings, Feeling Stronger, and Advanced Moves. If you are a complete newcomer to Pilates, start by assessing your posture and identifying any problems, then do the breathing exercises and make sure you've got the hang of them before attempting the "First Time" routine on page 184. Don't overdo it at your first session: 20 minutes is long enough, so do only a few repetitions of each of the exercises listed. If you can't manage one of them, stop and try another. Aim to do a Pilates session every second day, if you can. That way, your muscles will be well rested but they will "remember" how the movements felt from your previous session.

Devising a Program

Choose different sequences, focusing one day on the upper body, and another on the legs, pelvic area, or back. If you like, you can design your own routines to focus on your weakest parts. Every session should include abdominal curls, glute squeezes, hamstring curls, and pelvic tilts. Try to cover most areas, but choose two or three exercises that concentrate on the muscles you want to strengthen. Don't avoid the exercises you don't like or find difficult; they're probably the ones you need the most! If you have been working hard on a group of muscles, always remember to stretch them out afterward. Stay with the Gentle Beginnings routines (*pages 184–85*) until you can do ten controlled repetitions of all the exercises, then move onto Feeling Stronger (*pages 186–87*). You might want to work for up to 45 minutes in a session. When you can complete the Feeling Stronger programs, go to Advanced Moves (*pages 188–89*) and allow up to an hour per session.

Special cases

Children below the age of ten are unlikely to have the necessary concentration to take part in Pilates. Teenagers, however, should be encouraged to work on their posture, as they are growing fast and postural problems

Exercise balls
These are readily available by mail order.

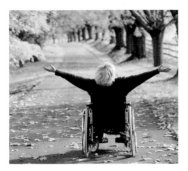

Wheelchair users
Most of the arm and upper torso exercises
can be done in a wheelchair, as can static
abs and several others.

WHEN TO EXERCISE

● Some people prefer to exercise in
the morning, while others like to wind
down at the end of the working day.
Choose a time that suits you, when you
won't be interrupted. Take the phone
off the hook and make sure family
members understand that you are not
to be disturbed.

● Don't exercise after a meal, when
you are ill, or if you are in pain or
taking painkillers.

can easily set in during this period. It's depressing to read news reports
about the number of children who never get any exercise. Pilates
teaches teenagers to take control of their own bodies and, with any
luck, they'll catch the exercise habit for life.

There is no upper age limit for Pilates. People in their 80s can be
more flexible than 30-year-olds. The great thing with older people who
take up Pilates, perhaps after years of never exercising, is that they will
see changes extremely quickly. They are generally more willing to work
hard and overcome any problems that have developed over the years.

If you are overweight and starting Pilates in combination with a
weight-loss diet, focus on building your core stability for the first few
weeks. Do some static abs, pelvic tilts, and gentle stretches every day.
Be honest about your flabby areas and concentrate on them. It will be
hard work, but the results will be worth it.

Even those with serious disabilities and mobility problems can
benefit from Pilates. There are several exercises you can do in a chair,
including static abs, sitting lats, arm exercises, and neck stretches.

Gentle Beginnings

Read through each exercise carefully before you try it so that you don't have to refer back to the directions. The pictures show a selection of movements from each of the routines, to act as a quick reminder. You may like to keep a notebook in which you list the exercises you've worked on in each session and the number of repetitions you managed. You'll be amazed how quickly you'll progress.

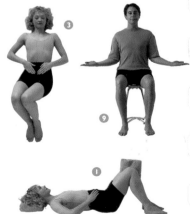

FIRST TIME

1   breathing with a scarf or towel (*page 32*)
2   static abs—lying on your side (*page 52*)
3   glute squeezes (*page 80*)
4   hamstring curls (*page 84*)
5   back stretches—stretch 1 (*page 112*)
6   pelvic tilts—stage 1 (*page 88*)
7   abdominal curls (*page 56*)
8   sitting lats (*page 108*)
9   crawling up the wall (*page 130*)
10   adductor cushion squeeze (*page 92*)

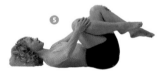

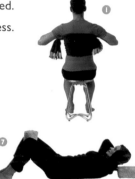

FOCUS ON THE PELVIS

1   static abs—semisupine (*page 53*)
2   pelvic tilts—stage 1 (*page 88*)
3   small hip rolls (*page 66*)
4   larger hip rolls (*page 68*)
5   abdominal curls (*page 56*)
6   glute squeezes (*page 80*)
7   hamstring curls (*page 84*)
8   back stretches—stretch 2 (*page 113*)
9   working the lats (*page 120*)
10   cossack arms (*page 122*)

FOCUS ON THE LEGS

1 glute squeezes (*page 80*)

2 hamstring curls (*page 84*)

3 pelvic tilts—stage 1 (*page 88*)

4 abdominal curls (*page 56*)

5 cross-fiber ab curls (*page 64*)

6 the Shell (*page 168*)

7 outer thighs—lying on side (*page 164*)

8 inner thighs—sitting (*page 162*)

9 working the lats—variation 1 (*page 121*)

10 working the lats—variation 2 (*page 121*)

FOCUS ON THE UPPER TORSO

1 breathing into your back (*page 35*)

2 sitting lats (*page 108*)

3 cossack arms (*page 122*)

4 side stretches (*page 132*)

5 glute squeezes (*page 80*)

6 hamstring curls (*page 84*)

7 the Arrow (*page 100*)

8 back stretches—stretch 2 (*page 113*)

9 pelvic tilts—stage 1 (*page 88*)

10 abdominal curls (*page 56*)

FOCUS ON THE BACK

1 breathing with a scarf or towel (*page 32*)

2 sitting lats—with a belt (*page 111*)

3 working the lats (*page 120*)

4 cossack arms (*page 122*)

5 the Arrow (*page 100*)

6 the Cobra (*page 72*)

7 pelvic tilts—stage 1 (*page 88*)

8 abdominal curls (*page 56*)

9 the Shake (*page 94*)

10 the Windmill (*page 124*)

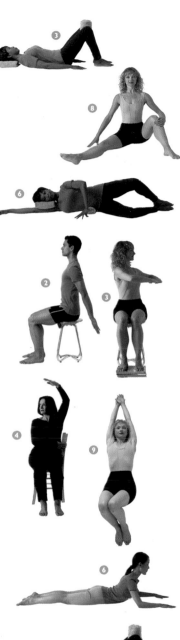

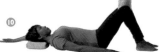

Feeling Stronger

From now on, when a routine lists abdominal curls, you should include cross-fiber curls as well to make sure all the abdominal muscles are worked. Pelvic tilts should start with the Stage I part, then go onto the stage that is recommended. Always do glute squeezes before hamstring curls at every session. These routines will take around 45 minutes to complete.

GENERAL EXERCISES

1 static abs (*page 52*)

2 pelvic tilts—stage 2 (*page 90*)

3 leg slides—sliding on a chair (*page 55*)

4 hip rolls—small and large (*pages 66–69*)

5 abdominal curls (*pages 56 and 64*)

6 the Shell (*page 168*)

7 hamstring curls (*page 84*)

8 inner thighs—sitting (*page 162*)

9 working the lats (*page 120*)

10 side stretches (*page 132*)

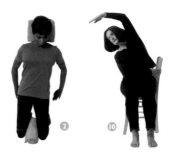

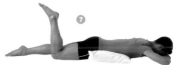

FOCUS ON CORE STABILITY

1 static abs (*page 52*)

2 single leg lifts (*page 54*)

3 pelvic tilts—stage 2 (*page 90*)

4 abdominal curls (*pages 56 and 64*)

5 upper torso release (*page 126*)

6 hamstring curls (*page 84*)

7 inner thighs—sitting (*page 162*)

8 sitting lats—with a belt (*page 111*)

9 hip rolls (*pages 66–69*)

10 the Shake (*page 94*)

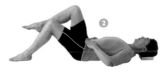

FOCUS ON THE LEGS

1 hamstring curls (*page 84*)
2 the Shell (*page 168*)
3 outer thighs—lying on side (*page 164*)
4 inner thighs—lying on side (*page 166*)
5 quadriceps (*page 170*)
6 leg stretches (*pages 176*)
7 pelvic tilts—stage 2 (*page 90*)
8 abdominal curls (*pages 56 and 64*)
9 crawling up the wall (*page 130*)
10 cossack arms (*page 122*)

FOCUS ON THE UPPER TORSO

1 sitting lats—variation 1 (*page 110*)
2 working the lats (*page 120*)
3 working the lats—variation 3 (*page 123*)
4 pillow squeezes (*page 136*)
5 cossack arms (*page 122*)
6 upper torso release (*page 126*)
7 the Windmill—making a circle (*page 125*)
8 hamstring curls (*page 84*)
9 the Arrow (*page 100*)
10 abdominal curls (*pages 56 and 64*)

FOCUS ON THE BACK

1 breathing into your back (*page 35*)
2 the Cat (*page 104*)
3 hamstring curls (*page 84*)
4 pelvic tilts—stage 2 (*page 90*)
5 the Star (*page 102*)
6 abdominal curls (*pages 56 and 64*)
7 the Cobra (*page 72*)
8 sitting lats—variation 2 (*page 111*)
9 cossack arms (*page 122*)
10 side stretches (*page 132*)

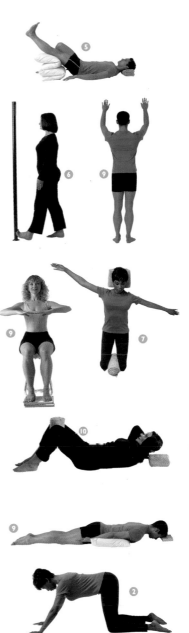

Advanced Moves

Don't try any of these routines until your core stability is good and you can manage the exercises in the Feeling Stronger section with confidence. If a movement feels uncomfortable, stop immediately, then check your position carefully and try again; if it still causes strain, leave it for now and go back to it in a few weeks. By now, you should be able to recognize the correct muscle movements for yourself.

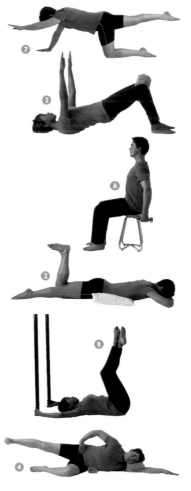

GENERAL EXERCISES

1. the Windmill—making a circle (*page 125*)
2. pelvic tilts—stages 1–3 (*pages 88–91*)
3. abdominal curls (*pages 56 and 64*)
4. hamstring curls (*page 84*)
5. the Arrow (*page 100*)
6. the Shell (*page 168*)
7. the Dog (*page 106*)
8. arm exercises (with weights) (*pages 152–57*)
9. side stretches—variation 1 (*page 133*)
10. neck stretches (*page 146*)

FOCUS ON CORE STABILITY

1. hamstring curls (*page 84*)
2. hamstring curls—variation 3 (*page 87*)
3. the Arrow (*page 100*)
4. outer thighs—lying on side (*page 164*)
5. inner thighs—lying on side (*page 166*)
6. double leg lifts (*page 165*)
7. pelvic tilts—stages 1–3 (*pages 88–91*)
8. reverse curls (*page 62*)
9. cross-fiber ab curls (*page 64*)
10. upper torso release (*pages 126*)

FOCUS ON THE LEGS

1 hamstring curls—variation 3 (*page 87*)

2 quadriceps—sitting on a table (*page 171*)

3 outer thighs—lying on side (*page 164*)

4 inner thighs—lying on side (*page 166*)

5 pelvic tilts—stages 1–3 (*pages 88–91*)

6 hip rolls (*pages 66–69*)

7 abdominal curls (*page 56*)

8 cross-fiber ab curls (*page 64*)

9 plié (*page 174*)

10 leg stretches (*page 176*)

FOCUS ON THE UPPER TORSO

1 sitting lats—variation 1 (*page 110*)

2 working the lats (*page 120*)

3 pillow squeezes (*page 136*)

4 upper torso release (*page 126*)

5 shoulder release (*page 128*)

6 crawling up the wall (*page 130*)

7 the Star (*page 102*)

8 the Cat (*page 104*)

9 pelvic tilts—stages 1–3 (*pages 88–91*)

10 abdominal curls (*pages 56 and 64*)

FOCUS ON THE BACK

1 pelvic tilts—stages 2 and 3 (*pages 90–91*)

2 abdominal curls (*page 56*)

3 cross-fiber ab curls (*page 64*)

4 large hip rolls—variation (*page 69*)

5 the Cobra (*page 72*)

6 hamstring curls (*page 84*)

7 the Star (*page 102*)

8 the Cat (*page 104*)

9 the Dog, and variation (*pages 106–7*)

10 side stretches—variation 2 (*page 133*)

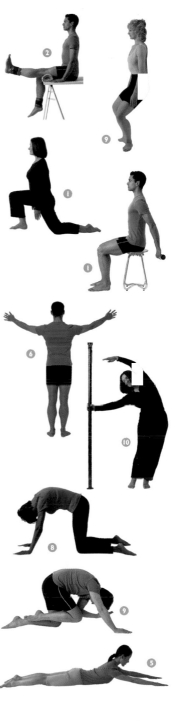

Pilates During Pregnancy

Dramatic changes occur to women's bodies during pregnancy, but Pilates can help them to adapt and avoid physical damage, while keeping in good shape for a healthy delivery. Even if you don't have any health problems, you should consult your physician before starting an exercise program while pregnant, and take it very gradually if you're not used to exercising. It is a good idea for women to learn Pilates before they become pregnant, to build their core stability first. If you are already pregnant, book a few sessions of one-to-one tuition to learn the techniques under supervision (*see page 203 for how to find your nearest studio*). It is advisable not to exercise during the first 12 weeks of pregnancy.

Fifty percent of women suffer back pain during pregnancy, and it's hardly surprising when you consider the extra strain being placed on the spine. The average weight gain is 22–31 pounds (10–14 kg) and most of this goes on the front of the body in the breasts and abdomen, so the center of gravity moves upward and forward. This causes the lower back to arch, while the shoulders pull forward and

TAKE CARE

Do not exercise during pregnancy if you have kidney, heart, or lung problems; diabetes; thyroid complaints; a history of miscarriage, premature labor, or cervical incompetence; vaginal bleeding; high blood pressure; a multiple pregnancy; an abnormal placenta; anemia; or if the baby is in the breech position after 28 weeks.

the neck arches back to counterbalance it
all. Every natural curve in the spine
is therefore exaggerated.

On top of this, hormones cause the
ligaments to soften and become more pliable,
making the joints weaker and more
vulnerable. The abdominal muscles are
weakened as they are progressively stretched
and, from about six months, the rectus
abdominis muscle can separate down the
middle, making the abdominals work even less
efficiently. For all these reasons, strenuous,
high-impact exercises are not advised during
pregnancy; weight-training can be dangerous,
and anything that involves rapid, jerky
movements could damage your joints.

By working the muscles that promote
core stability during midpregnancy, you will
be more stable in later stages and suffer fewer
joint and muscular aches and pains. You are
also less likely to get breathless in late
pregnancy if you've kept the alignment of your
upper spine correct. However, there are some
positions and movements that you should
avoid at different stages, so read through
this section carefully before you begin.

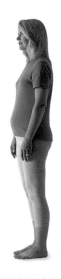

Correct posture
It is easier to maintain
good posture if your
core stability muscles
are already strong.

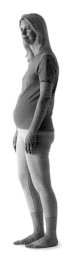

Incorrect posture
The extra weight in front
of your body can cause the
curves of the spine to
become exaggerated.

Pilates During Pregnancy

Posture and Breathing

All the normal postural rules apply when you are pregnant. Always stand with your chin level and held slightly back so that your neck is straight; keep your shoulders level and don't let them hunch forward; contract your abdominal muscles to support the lower spine; soften your knees so that your weight is balanced over the center of each foot. Follow the advice given on page 23 when sitting, and avoid lifting heavy weights altogether. Pilates breathing exercises can be extremely helpful during labor and are a great way to help you relax and release tension. It is especially important to breathe correctly while exercising to facilitate the movements and avoid straining your upper spine.

PREGNANCY CHECKLIST

Avoid:
- Any high-impact exercises with rapid, jerky movements
- Any exercise that involves full flexion or extension of the joints
- Deep stretching or resistance exercises using weights
- Any form of exercise that raises your heartbeat above 140 beats per minute
- Lying on your front once you have a "bump"

After 30 weeks, avoid:
- Lying on your back
- Any movements that abduct your hips

Always:
- Stop immediately if you feel tired or experience any pain or discomfort
- Check with your doctor before starting an exercise program while pregnant

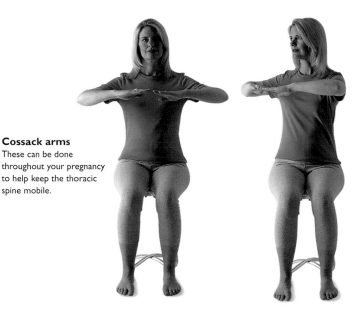

Cossack arms
These can be done throughout your pregnancy to help keep the thoracic spine mobile.

The abdominals

Strong abdominals will help you maintain good posture and support your spine. Focus on repetitions of static abs, rather than ab curls. If the rectus abdominus muscle separates at around six months, you can still use the transverse abdominals. This will minimize the separation and help it to close up more quickly after the birth. After 30 weeks, you should avoid lying on your back, as there is a slight risk of a blood vessel called the inferior vena cava becoming compressed, but you can still pull your navel back while lying on your side or on all fours (see *page 51*).

The pelvic area

Pelvic floor exercises are encouraged throughout pregnancy and the postnatal period, as these muscles can stretch and weaken with the weight of the uterus and during vaginal deliveries. Try to do 50

squeezes every day. Glute squeezes and small pelvic tilts are great
for maintaining pelvic stability and stretching the lower back muscles.
After it becomes uncomfortable to lie on your front, keep doing
standing and sitting glute squeezes. In later pregnancy, when the pelvic
ligaments are especially soft, avoid movements that abduct your hip
(move it outward). When climbing out of bed or getting out of a car,
don't stretch outward with one leg; swivel your hips around instead,
keeping your legs close together. Avoid swimming breaststroke or
squatting, which both abduct the hip.

The back

The Cat and Dog (*pages 104–7*) are safe throughout pregnancy
and will help to relieve any back pain. You can also do sitting lats
(*see page 108*) and pillow squeezes (*see page 136*) throughout, but
avoid the Arrow and the Star (*see pages 100–3*) when it becomes
uncomfortable to lie on your front. The Alexander rest (*see page
114*) is great for relaxation. After 30 weeks, you can do it lying on
your side. Put a small cushion between your legs and another one
under your bump. Make sure your head is comfortably supported
and then breathe deeply, feeling your muscles relax into the floor.

The exercises for the Upper Torso, Neck, and Shoulders are
all extremely beneficial throughout pregnancy, although you should
avoid any that involve lying on your back after 30 weeks. The exercises
for the lats are particularly good for strengthening the middle of your
back, but do them without weights. You can try the Windmill
standing up in late pregnancy.

The legs and feet

The extra weight you are carrying puts a lot of strain on your legs and feet, but by keeping the muscles strong and the circulation good you can avoid classic pregnancy complaints such as swollen ankles, varicose veins, and painful arches. Calf raises are good for relieving cramp, and you should dome your feet whenever you have a spare moment. Remember to avoid any movements in late pregnancy that abduct your hips: the Shell (*see page 168*) and the adduction and abduction exercises on pages 162–67 would not be suitable after 30 weeks. Hamstring stretches can be done in a sitting position after 30 weeks: sitting straight, loop a scarf or towel around one foot and straighten the leg, keeping the other leg bent. Lean forward from the hips while pulling your leg up with the towel, and feel the stretch. Put your feet up, then point and flex them to help the circulation in your calves and ankles.

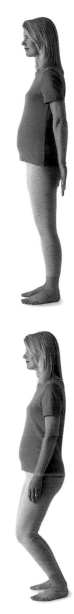

Pliés
These are good for strengthening the legs, but stop doing them after 30 weeks.

PREGNANCY ROUTINES

12–30 weeks

1 elbow circles (*page 118*)
2 arm circles (*page 119*)
3 calf raises (*page 173*)
4 spine roll-down (*page 24*)
5 static abs—lying on your side (*page 52*)
6 leg slides—sliding on a chair (*page 55*)
7 leg stretches (*pages 176–79*)
8 sitting lats—variation 2 (*page 11*)
9 the Windmill (*page 124*)
10 Alexander rest (*page 114*)

30 weeks and onward

1 static abs on all fours (*page 51*)
2 the Cat—steps 1 and 2 only (*page 104*)
3 the Dog (*page 106*)
4 back stretch—stretch 2 (*page 113*)
5 calf raises (*page 173*)
6 quadriceps—sitting on a table (*page 171*)
7 hamstring stretches, sitting up (*page 177*)
8 sitting lats (*page 108*)
9 elbow circles (*page 118*)
10 Alexander rest on your side (*page 114*)

Lower leg exercises

This is good for relaxing the legs, and
exercising the calves and feet. If you don't
have an exercise ball, lie on the floor
and rest your leg on a sofa or chair that
is the correct height.

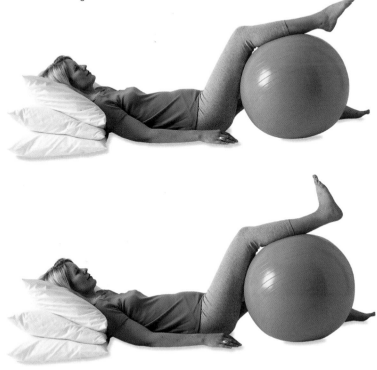

Static abs
These should be done lying on your side
after 30 weeks.

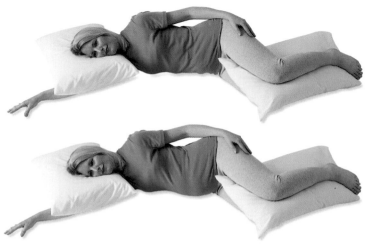

The postnatal period

It can take up to six months for the ligaments supporting your joints

to return to their prepregnancy state, and even longer if you are still

breast-feeding. It is crucial that you continue to follow the postural

advice, especially when lifting and carrying your baby. Use cushions to

make sure you are well supported and not hunching your shoulders

forward when feeding. Avoid heavy lifting or straining until you can hold

your pelvic floor exercises for ten seconds at a time, or you could risk

vaginal prolapse or stress incontinence. Keep doing static abs to

reinforce core stability, and add in a few small pelvic tilts.

Women who have had a cesarian section will recover around six

weeks later than those who delivered vaginally, but you will be able

to start pulling your navel to your spine soon after your cesarian.

Avoid exercises that involve kneeling on all fours until you have

passed your six-week checkup.

Pilates for Life

Get into the habit of doing your Pilates workouts every second day—or as often as you can manage. At the same time, you should be thinking about your posture throughout your daily activities, and correcting it when necessary. Always stand with your hips square and your weight balanced through your feet. Sit straight with your shoulders back and shoulderblades down. Use the whole of your lungs to breathe. Maintain an awareness of your abdominal muscles when sitting or standing.

Daily Pilates

Certain Pilates exercises can be incorporated into your daily routine:

● While sitting in the car, pull your navel to your spine and do some glute squeezes

● Standing at the kitchen sink, do some calf raises and standing glute squeezes

● While in the office, do some sitting lats, Cossack arms, and side stretches, and dome your feet

● At any time of day, do your pelvic floor exercises. No one will ever guess!

If you have a spare 10 or 15 minutes, do a mini-routine of four or five exercises. You should also do some kind of aerobic exercise on a regular basis. Choose something you enjoy, which gets your heart rate up: tennis, running, cycling, swimming, rock climbing—the choice is yours. Use your knowledge of the way the muscles work to ensure you exercise safely, without putting undue stress on your joints. Always warm up beforehand and do some stretches afterward. You can do aerobic exercise on a day when you're not doing a Pilates session, or use a Gentle Beginnings workout as your warm-up.

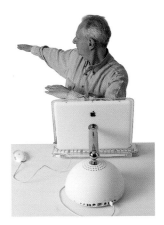

Cossack arms
Good for releasing upper back tension when sitting at a computer.

If you've worked through the exercises in this book and would like to learn more about Pilates, see the details on page 203 on how to find a local studio or matwork class. In Pilates studios, you will do many of the exercises we've covered here, but you'll be working on weight machines that use springs to provide resistance. The body is held in the correct position while the muscles work to a higher intensity. Trained staff will show you how the machines are set up and supervise you as you exercise. Make sure the studio you choose has a good range of machines, that it is not overcrowded, and that there is at least one member of staff to every four clients.

When choosing a matwork class, make sure there are no more than eight pupils at a time. Watch a class first to see how much supervision is given, and have a chat with the teacher. They should take details of any injuries or weaknesses, along with a general medical history. Some classes are aimed at beginners while others are more advanced, so discuss which would be best for you.

Motivation

The most difficult clients to teach are the ones who come into a Pilates studio and expect the teacher to do all the work for them. It seems that they are looking for an easy answer and are not prepared to do what it takes to make changes. Exercise—even Pilates—is not the most exciting part of life, but it's essential for good health. It should be seen as part of your routine, like cleaning your teeth: not the best fun, but we all have to do it.

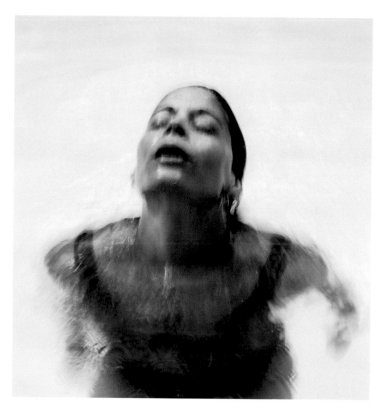

Swimming
If you are swimming, make sure you have learned the strokes correctly and are not straining your back by holding your head up out of the water.

Everyday Pilates
Is she doing her glute squeezes or her pelvic floors as she washes the dishes? Who can tell!

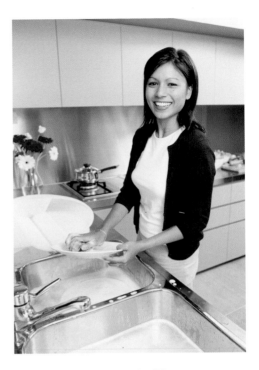

Having said that, the vast majority of people learning Pilates are very enthusiastic and dedicated. They're excited by the physical changes they can see and feel, and are determined to get better and better. After the very first session, you'll feel looser and more relaxed, and the benefits are only just beginning.

Remember what Joseph Pilates said? Within 10 sessions you'll feel better; if you're exercising every second day, that's in only three weeks' time. Within 20 sessions (six weeks) you'll see the difference and after 30 sessions (nine weeks) you'll have a whole new body. Why not get your diary out and make a mark three, six, and nine weeks from today, to remind you how quickly you can make changes.

Now, take the phone off the hook and start your first Pilates workout. Good luck!

Questions & Answers

 I'm 65 years old and I've never exercised in my life. Isn't it too late to start?

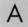 No! It's never too late. Go slowly and you'll be amazed how much your muscles will respond. Check with your physician before starting, just to be on the safe side.

 I had been doing Pilates for two years, then I lapsed and haven't done anything for the last six months. Do I have to start with Gentle Beginnings again?

 Just do a few Gentle Beginnings sessions to remind the body how it was working before, then pick the level you feel confident with. If you did Pilates for two years, then you should still have good core stability even after a six-month break.

Which exercises shall I show my 10-year-old daughter first? Should I do all the Gentle Beginnings routines with her?

It depends what she needs. If she has postural problems, teach her to sit, stand, and carry her schoolbag correctly, then work on simple core stability exercises such as ab curls, small pelvic tilts, glute squeezes, and hamstring curls. If she gets tension in her shoulders, check her posture and show her the Windmill and shoulder release exercises.

Are there any Pilates exercises I can do while watching television?

Yes, you could do static abs, pelvic floors, and foot doming, but that's all. Other Pilates exercises require you to concentrate on the movements and the feeling in your muscles, and that's not possible with a TV blaring in the background.

Useful Addresses

There are so many Pilates studios
in the US that it would be
impossible to list them all here. A
company called Balanced Body
keeps a full listing, which you can
use to find your nearest studio.

Contact them on:
E-mail: info@pilates.com
Website: www.pilates.com
Tel: (916) 388 2838, (800) 745 2837
Fax: (916) 379 9277
Address: 8220 Ferguson Avenue,
Sacramento, CA 95828-0931

If you want to contact
Alan Herdman, you can write
to him at:
Alan Herdman Studios
17 Homer Row
London W1H 4AP
UK

Glossary

For descriptions of the position and function of individual muscles, see pages 42–45.

Abduction
A movement that draws away from the central line of the body. In the outer thigh abduction exercises, the legs are moved outward to the side. The muscles that carry out this movement are known as abductors.

Adduction
A movement toward the central line of the body. In the inner thigh adduction exercises, the legs are moved inward, and the muscles that carry out the movement are known as adductors.

Core stability
Strong muscles in the body's center of gravity, between the base of the ribs and the pelvis, that help to align and balance the body while protecting the spine. Achieving core stability is a fundamental aim of Pilates.

Engaging muscles
Bringing them into operation. When you are asked to engage the abdominals, it means pulling your navel back toward your spine. To engage the lats, pull your shoulderblades down slightly.

Exercise ball
A large ball used for some Pilates exercises. Available in many stores or by mail order.

Extension
Lengthening out or straightening. If you are asked to extend your arm, you should straighten a bent elbow.

Flexion
Bending or folding. Flexor muscles are responsible for bending your fingers, for example.

Glutes
Our shorthand for the gluteus maximus muscles across the buttocks. glute squeezes work these muscles.

Hamstrings
A group of muscles at the back of the thigh, which bend the knee and swing the leg backward from the thigh.

Isometric

A movement that contracts a muscle without shortening it. See, for example, the isometric neck exercises on page 144.

Kyphosis

An excessive forward curve of the upper (thoracic) spine. See page 20.

Lats

Our shorthand for the latissimus dorsi muscle in the middle of the back, which moves the arm downward and backward.

Ligament

A tough band of slightly elastic tissue that holds bones together at joints and prevents the joints from moving too far.

Lordosis

A pronounced inward curve in the lower (lumbar) spine. See page 19.

Prone

Lying on your front.

Quads

Our shorthand for the quadriceps muscles at the front of the thigh, which are responsible for straightening the knee.

Rotation

Movement around a central axis. If you are asked to rotate the upper body around the spine, the spine should stay straight. An inward rotation of the leg would mean that the heel faced outward.

Scoliosis

A condition in which the spine is bent to one side in the upper (thoracic) or lower (lumbar) area or both. See page 19.

Semisupine

A common position for Pilates exercises, in which you lie on your back with your knees bent.

Soft

When joints are "soft," they are slightly bent and not locked. There should be no tension in a soft joint.

Index

ACKNOWLEDGMENTS

Hair, makeup, and styling: Richard Burns

Models
Clovissa Newcombe, Sara Gallie, Grace Grosvenor, Reiko Muira, Joshua Tuifua,
Peter Ottevanger, Harry Ditson, Jennifer Rhule

Photo Credits
The publisher would like to thank the following for the use of images:

Corbis Joyce Choo 201 / Jon Feingersh 183 / Ken Kaminesky 77

Imagebank Peter Cade 76 / Ghislain & Marie David de Lossy 118tl /
Michelangelo Gratton 18 / Pink Fridge Productions 30

Taxi Ericka McConnell 50tr / V.C.L 21 / Christopher Wilhelm 31b

Photo of Alan Herdman, page 6, by Gemma Levine

Photo of Joseph Pilates, page 9, by I.C. Rapaport